The Patient in the Family

The Patient in the Family

An Ethics of Medicine and Families

Hilde Lindemann Nelson
and James Lindemann Nelson

Routledge
New York and London

Published in 1995 by

Routledge
29 West 35 Street
New York, NY 10001

Published in Great Britain in 1995 by

Routledge
11 New Fetter Lane
London EC4P 4EE

Library of Congress Cataloging-in-Publications Data

Nelson, Hilde Lindemann.
    The Patient in the Family : an ethics of medicine and families / by Hilde Lindemann Nelson
    and James Lindemann Nelson.
        p.   cm.
    Includes bibliographical references and notes.
    ISBN 0–415–91128–1 (cl.) — ISBN 0–415–91129–X (pbk.)
    1. Medical ethics. 2. Family. 3. Family medicine. I. Nelson, James Lindemann. II. Title.
        [DNLM: 1. Ethics, Medical. 2. Family Health. 3. Family—psychology.
    4. Professional–Family Relations. W 50 N426p 1995]
    R724.N43 1995
    174'.2—dc20
    DNLM/DLC   94–33652
    for Library of Congress   CIP

iiii

This book is for

ELISE ROBINSON
ELLEN ROBINSON
ERIC NELSON
PAUL ROBINSON
LAURA NELSON
MELISSA NELSON

Contents

Preface

WHEN SOMEONE IS SICK OR PREGNANT OR BEGINNING TO UNDERGO THE ravages of old age, it seems perfectly natural to look to the institution of medicine for care. It's less apparent that another institution, even older than medicine, continues to provide care for millions of Americans, sometimes in cooperation with the health care system and sometimes in lieu of it. This second institution is that of the family, and the health services it provides range from tea and sympathy when Dad has the flu, to years of care for a son or daughter suffering from schizophrenia, to live donation of a lung or liver lobe for a family member who will die without it.

Increasingly, these two systems of care are rubbing each other the wrong way. Families make unreasonable demands on the health care system when they expect it to perform high-tech miracles that will cure everything from midlife crises to death itself. Medicine makes unreasonable demands on families when its reproductive technologies lure subfertile couples into yet another attempt at in vitro fertilization, at $10,000 a pop, or when new fetal surgery techniques up the ante for the kinds of sacrifices that pregnant women are expected to undergo.

The problem is a serious one and may soon reach alarming proportions. It has already created a climate of mutual mistrust and suspicion, in which doctors are tempted to practice defensive medicine for fear of being sued for malpractice, while families, already buffeted by a high divorce rate, inadequate social services, and fewer women at home to look after the young and infirm, are showing signs of cracking under the strain. Set all this in an era of rising health insurance premiums and runaway medical inflation, a growing pessimism about whether physicians really have a patient's interests at heart, and a similar pessimism about how abusive families really are and have always been, and you have the makings of a first-class crisis.

We see this crisis as fundamentally a moral or ethical one (we use these terms interchangeably throughout the book). Therefore, when we ask, "What can be done to reduce the friction between medicine and families? How can the two systems of care come to understand one another better so that they can help rather than hinder the other's efforts to perform its proper functions?" we take it that we're raising questions of ethics, rather than of policy or law. As we thought about them it struck us that, while an exploration of the ethics by which the medical profession operates has become a major smokeless industry in the last quarter of a century, far less attention has been paid to the ethics of families. They too have their code of conscience, and even the most casual glance reveals that it is quite different from the code of the physician.

It is the task of this book to examine the difference, particularly as it plays itself out in the clinic and at the bedside. Our strategy has been, first, to set the two systems in their historical context, so we could get some sense of how they arrived at their present pass. Then we devoted some attention to the question of why families matter, given current levels of dissatisfaction with them and even scattered calls to abolish them altogether. Having done that, we were ready to explore the morally significant features of medicine and families, with an eye to understanding how and why they differ. These questions occupy the first three chapters. Once we had identified these features in a general way, we were ready to put them to work on specific areas of interaction between medicine and families. Chapter Four is devoted to the role of families in medical decisionmaking; Chapter Five discusses families' involvement in the care of the elderly; Chapter Six considers the stake of families in the new reproductive technologies. And in Chapter Seven we examine the demands for social justice that have only now begun to upset the health care system, some twenty-five years after the women's movement began to demand justice within families.

The history of health care in the United States has been quite different from that of its European or Canadian counterparts, to say nothing of that of southern countries. American families too carry their own distinctive stamp. For that reason, we've confined our discussion to the way the two systems of care pull against each other in the United States, recognizing full well that the dynamics may be quite different in other countries.

Our work bears the stamp of professional and domestic experience. Our professional home is the Hastings Center, an institute where scholars reflect carefully and systematically on how to resolve the tensions in our values caused by biomedical advances. Our familial home contains (when we're lucky) our six children, aged thirteen to twenty-three. Blending us all into a new family once posed its own tensions and complexities, which required no less careful reflection.

It's our hope that the insights of this book will go some distance toward easing the growing friction between families and medicine. But if that hope is to pan out, the book must speak clearly to two audiences: professionals in health care and ethics, and members of families, whatever their occupation. Health care givers and ethicists who work with them are doing their best in a medical system that has grown not only technically but also morally puzzling and deeply complex: this book is offered to them. Primarily, however, it is addressed to those who enter hospitals, nursing homes, and doctor's offices through other doors—as patients and worried family members trying to care for someone they love. To our friends and teachers in both groups our deepest gratitude; this book could not have been written without them.

In addition to these general sentiments, we can't deny ourselves the pleasure of thanking some people in particular. For assistance with research we drew upon the talents of Eric Nelson and Paul Robinson (who are even more satisfying as sons), and Julie Rothstein, a very dear friend. Several physicians were particularly generous with their insights; we thank

Dr. Joseph Jack Fins, Dr. Willard Gaylin, Dr. Joanne Lynn, and, most especially, Dr. Lainie Freedman Ross. Professor Martha Blauvelt tried to gently direct our enthusiasm as amateur historians. Philosophers and theologians to whom we owe special gratitude are Jeffrey Blustein, Philip Boyle, John Hardwig, Richard T. Hull, Erik Parens, Sara Ruddick, William Ruddick, and Susan Sherwin. And finally, heartfelt thanks to Daniel Callahan, the founder of the feast.

Chapter One

A Rivalry of Care

iĺiii

A LITTLE GIRL IS SUFFERING FROM KIDNEY FAILURE. The physical, emotional and social burdens of her thrice-weekly, six-hour long sessions on the dialysis machine are becoming harder and harder for her to bear. Her doctors aren't sure a kidney transplant would work—she has already rejected one cadaver kidney—but they are willing to try it, if they can find a biologically compatible donor. The pediatrician privately tells the father that he is compatible. How can he possibly say no? Yet he does. It isn't just that the outcome is so uncertain—he is frightened of the operation itself, and of what will happen to him and his other two children if the remaining kidney ever gave out. Ashamed to refuse, he asks the physician to tell the family that he isn't a good match. The pediatrician, despite her sympathy, says she can't lie for him. There is a long silence. "Okay, then. I'll give her my kidney. If they knew I could but I wouldn't, it'd wreck the family."[1]

Why would it wreck the family? Does a father have a special obligation to donate a kidney to his suffering daughter? What is it about families that arouses such strong expectations that parents will sacrifice themselves for their children? And what is it about medicine that amplifies, distorts, transforms those expectations?

A gray-haired woman lies stretched on a delivery table. She's not having a particularly easy time of it. Now in her mid-forties, it's been twenty years since she last gave birth. On that occasion, she had a little girl, perfect in all but one respect—the child was born without a uterus. This time, the baby who is about to be born grew from her daughter's egg and her son-in-law's sperm, united in a Petrie dish, and then implanted into her womb.

While many mothers have not been birthgivers, for the whole history of our species, we have regarded all birthgivers as mothers: in its core meaning, a "mother" is a woman from whose body a child issues. But despite her birth pains, this middle-aged woman does not think of herself as mother to the child she is bearing. Medicine's ability to fertilize eggs in vitro allows her to think of herself as the grandmother, instead. But what happens if she comes to believe she's the child's mother after all? *Should* she believe this? What will the child think when he grows up? Will this use of medical technology affect not just this woman, this child, and their family, but how all of us think and feel about our most intimate ties?

Cases like these were once utterly impossible, then exceedingly rare. Now they are becoming a part of the everyday landscape of our lives. Two of our most valued and most influential social institutions—the family and medicine—are grinding against each other like glaciers, altering each other and the ground they traverse, but in ways we're only starting to notice, and with consequences whose outlines we're only beginning to trace.

In order better to see and evaluate just what's going on here, we need to understand the sometimes subtle, yet deeply significant, differences in the values that tend to prevail in families, on the one hand, and in medicine on the other. To get a sense of these differences, we needn't examine only high-tech or heroic cases; quite ordinary instances of day-to-day medical decisionmaking will do nicely. Consider a run-of-the-mill case of medical decisionmaking. The doctor weighs the merits of a given medical procedure solely in terms of benefits and risks to the patient, quite apart from any impact on other people. By this focus on the patient's interests alone, the patient—who is typically in a highly vulnerable position—is protected from arrogant misuse of the physician's power, and her significance as an individual person is affirmed. Yet if we step back from the doctor-patient dyad, and take seriously the fact that most patients are part of a family, this intensely single-minded focus will look rather odd. Is there any other area of human life where individual interests enjoy such a privileged position? Anything from changing careers to arranging an overnight business trip is ordinarily done in consultation with one's spouse or other intimates, since these people have a legitimate interest in the outcome.[2] In medicine, the patient alone is presumed to have an interest—a power to veto or demand that is categorically different from anyone else's, no matter how deeply others are affected by the decision.

The man who was afraid to donate his kidney thought he had failed his daughter because he wasn't willing to do everything he could to try to save her life; he thought he was being cowardly and a bad father. And perhaps he was. But another possibility he hadn't considered was that he was adopting the morality of medicine rather than honoring what's valuable about families. Both the father and the physicians believed that the only legitimate question here was, "What is in the best interest of the patient?" Yet families are made up of a number of people, all of whose interests have to be honored. The single focus on one individual may be fine for medicine, but it's less fine for families, who have their own, very different, mechanisms for protecting their vulnerable members. In times of illness, families—anxious, needy, and easily swayed—are drawn into medicine's overwhelming commitment to patient welfare. Family members lose sight of the value of family life at these times because, like a fish who takes water for granted, they generally live within such values without being explicitly aware of it.

In any case, family values are not well understood. It's easy not to notice that they differ from the values of medicine. Yet when families adopt the ethics of a rival system of care at times of greatest stress—at birth, death, disability, or illness—their members may unwittingly trample on the intricate web of relationships of which families are woven. This upsets the delicate balance between loving intimacy and individual growth that family members must continually maintain: too intense an intimacy is stifling and oppressive, yet, with too much distance, families become a mere aggregate of strangers. The balance is hard enough to maintain under the best of circumstances, but when a family is in trouble it becomes even harder.

The father's dilemma regarding kidney donation is compounded further. Nobody gave any thought to the fact that the choice he was forced to make could only occur within a very sophisticated setting: a modern organ transplantation center. It's one thing to do everything you can for someone you love when "everything" means arranging for an appendectomy and then staying with the patient as much as possible while she's recovering. It's quite another to be confronted with the technology of organ transplants, in which the economic, emotional, and physical costs of doing "everything" have undergone a quantum leap.

If medicine's characteristic focus on the good of the individual patient has distorted the way families interact with their sick members, so too have certain family values put pressure on medicine's own precarious understanding of itself, of its own deepest values and sense of mission. When medicine's basic offerings—the preservation of life, the cure of illness, and the ease of suffering—are unavailable to so many, we need to ask whether a subfertile couple's desire to found a family is really best seen as a medical problem, and whether the amount of resources devoted, say, to uniting eggs and sperm outside human bodies is well directed. Moreover, family pressure can increase doctors' confusions about their newfound power to keep bodies organically alive when all hope of life beyond the merely organic is gone. No longer unanimously convinced that their mandate is to preserve human life at whatever level of functioning, physicians have begun to regard sustaining the irreversibly comatose or the persistently vegetative as futile—a waste of medical resources, an affront to professional integrity. However, maintaining this sort of integrity becomes very difficult when families, driven by their own ideas of doing "everything," plead for therapy that physicians regard as bad medicine.

Medicine is being nudged into a form that may well be foreign to its own deepest traditions, but it pushes back even harder against families. A mother may undergo the rigors of pregnancy out of love for her daughter; what could seem a greater testimony to the significance of family bonds than that? But what is now a rare expression of motherly devotion might well be transformed through medical technology into something *expected* of women in such a situation. The father described above found that donating a kidney to his daughter is now perceived as a matter of basic decency. Will a similar standard of sacrifice come to govern the mother whose infertile daughter wants a child? And, as medicine has developed the means to extend the human lifespan by several decades,

4

but in the process merely prolonging, but not eradicating, the ills of old age, will family members now be expected to care for their frail and perhaps demented elderly relatives for many years? American families have traditionally looked after their old, but the weight of that care has become heavier and bids fair to last longer. Will families be expected as a matter of course to shoulder this greater burden?

Whether the need is for assistance with reproduction, cure of the sick, or care for the dying, the ends of medicine have subtly been altered by the pressure that families put on health care workers. Conversely, medicine's response may inadvertently damage significant features of family life, simply because its own values tend to obscure them. And because families, too, have failed fully to understand what is uniquely valuable about themselves, they may founder and are sometimes damaged through their interactions with a health care system that means them no harm in the world.

Given the importance of both systems of care in our lives, a *laissez-faire* approach to their relationship is not responsible. What we must have is informed and careful deliberation about what we want to preserve and what we need to change in both these institutions. To that end, we must develop an understanding, deeper than the "bioethics revolution" of the last twenty-five years has yet achieved, of what is morally important about both systems. A crucial means of gaining such understanding is to learn just how the conflict between them escalated to its present point. Before we do anything else, then, we need to trace the history in this country of the development of the family and the development of medicine.

In the rest of this chapter, we examine how social and technological changes have progressively led families to relinquish more and more of their traditional responsibility for health care to an increasingly powerful profession. We note how medicine was shaped by family needs, as well as by other forces that gave it its present technological and corporate character. We also note an important shift in the understanding of what makes families valuable—a shift to a child-centered, sentimental ideal of family life—and how as a result the family became more vulnerable to medical pressure. In later chapters, we explain certain enduring patterns in the histories of both institutions, and try to determine how these rivals can resolve their differences and become the allies we need them to be.

American Medicine and American Families before the Revolution

How did we come to our present pass? Why is it suddenly so much harder for these two systems of care to function smoothly together? To ask the question in this way suggests that medicine and families have always been distinct, yet this is not the case. For much of American history, the only health care available to most families was what they were able to provide for themselves. Medicine has been transformed in the last two centuries from a traditional profession with little relevance to ordinary households to a bureaucratic and corporate power on which families depend heavily.[3] Families during that same period exchanged a certain amount of social and economic autonomy for dependence on other institutions—including corporate medicine—as they increased their standard of living.[4] Social, scientific, and cultural change has thus brought families and medicine together, but has activated and magnified the latent tension between the values of families and those of physicians.

When Europeans first came to colonize the New World, the family was the natural source of care for the sick, and within the family such care fell to women. They were responsible for diagnosis, treatment, and nursing, as well as for putting up medicinal herbs along with the other preserves. Education in domestic medicine was acquired orally, from older women in the family or from neighbors, but also from native Americans, who taught the settlers the properties of unfamiliar plants and their own traditions of healing.

Later, in the colonial period, healing the sick and caring for the dying was still the responsibility of the adult women in the household. For those who could read, help was available from guidebooks written by physicians (who tended to be critical of the medical profession), in accessible language that avoided Latin or technical terms. The most popular of them, William Buchan's *Domestic Medicine*, was published in 1769 in Edinburgh and two years later in Philadelphia. Originally subtitled "an attempt to render the Medical Art more generally useful, by showing people what is in their own power both with respect to the Prevention and Cure of Diseases," it was reprinted at least thirty times and remained influential throughout the first half of the nineteenth century.

The publication of this and other populist physicians' guides was the mark of a profession struggling with its own identity. In eighteenth-century England—the fountainhead of the colonial professions—physicians were an elite, learned in the Latin and Greek that formed the core of a university education. Being gentlemen, physicians did not work with their hands as the barber-surgeons did, nor did they ply a trade, like the apothecaries. Rather, they developed theories of illness, based their diagnoses on them, and prescribed remedies. Their patients were members of the aristocracy, whose patronage they courted. In America, however, a society with a rhetoric of obliviousness to class distinctions, a gentrified physicianry was ill-suited to the revolutionary climate. If all men were created equal, how could a medical aristocracy be justified? Benjamin Rush, a signer of the Declaration of Independence and a major influence on American professional medicine through his teaching post at the University of Pennsylvania, counseled his students that upper-class affectation was "incompatible with the simplicity of science, and the real dignity of physic."[5]

Yet for all his republican politics and manners, Rush practiced a medicine that was as far removed from populist, domestic medicine as it could possibly be. His therapies were so dangerous that they could not safely be put into lay hands, and, for their day, they were high-technology, aggressive interventions. Rush believed that all disease had one cause—"morbid excitement induced by capillary tension"—and that the one remedy was therefore to deplete the body of its fluids. This he did by bloodletting with a lancet or with leeches, and by emptying the stomach and bowels with powerful drugs. Patients could be bled until they fainted, and were given heavy doses of mercurous chloride as a cathartic. Heroic therapy of this kind dominated professional medicine in the first few decades of the nineteenth century.

A backlash was bound to develop, not only because physicians' medicine was so dangerous, but also because in the Jacksonian era populist democratic attitudes pervaded all spheres of American life, including that of health care. The lay medicine that arose was not merely a substitute for professional medicine, but an active rival to it, closely allied to the medicine of families. Botanic practitioners and midwives were the most numerous lay health care workers, but native American doctors were also held in high esteem, as were bonesetters like the Sweet family of Rhode Island, who passed on their craft from one generation to the next between the seventeenth and the early twentieth century.

Postcolonial Developments:
Domestic Medicine and the Family of Sentiment

American families have always been somewhat fragile and subject to rapid reconfigurations. Early European observers noted that in the matrilineal Iroquois societies of the seventeenth century, to take only one instance, divorce was a common practice. Families in the Chesapeake colonies of Virginia and Maryland were so vulnerable to malaria and other fatal illnesses that it was not at all unusual for an adult, whether slave or free, to bury three or even four spouses, or for half-orphaned children—George Washington among them—to be reared by relatives other than the surviving parent. This fragility, however, did not keep the colonial family from being the primary economic and social unit, the producer of goods and services.

Between 1770 and 1830 a new kind of middle-class family came into existence. Like the colonial one, it was subject to reconfiguration through death, adoption, and remarriage, but it was marked by an increasing privacy, comfort, and child-centeredness. The shift was made possible in part by the fact that the material conditions of American life grew easier, in part also by a movement in European culture: a new emphasis on moral "sentiment" as a source of individual and social virtue. Intellectuals and artists in eighteenth-century Germany, France, and England became skeptical of the idea that morality was the embodiment of reason. Instead, they promoted the idea of the "man of sentiment," who honored his feelings and allowed them interplay with his intellect. Indeed, the philosopher David Hume inverted the earlier order: in practical matters, he declared, "Reason is, and ought only to be the slave of the passions, and can never pretend to any other office than to serve and obey them."[6] The newly invented novel, the French *comèdie larmoyante* (tearful comedy), and a spate of plays including Colley Cibber's *Careless Husband* and George Farquhar's *Recruiting Officer*, were called sentimental because their ideas were expressed in "sentiments"—statements of elevated and thoughtful feeling.

The new respect for the emotions was a part of the larger, Enlightenment idea of the importance of the individual. Individualism found a particularly warm welcome in America, where freedom was the watchword and the right of citizens to noninterference from the state (although not extended to slaves or free women) was prized highly. Self-reliance had been an

American virtue a hundred years before Emerson wrote on the subject in 1841. The idea of individual autonomy, coupled with the new understanding of the importance of feeling, produced a more democratic ideal of domestic life: that of a conjugal bond emphasizing companionship and affection, respect for each individual family member, and an intensified interest in children's upbringing and well-being.

The shift in sensibility was accompanied by a shift in gender roles. The father was to be the family's breadwinner, his workplace (in the Northeast, at any rate) less typically the farm or household than the counting houses, mills, shops, factories, and offices of urban life, where he was paid a wage for a clearly demarcated working day. His sphere of activity was the public sector. The mother's sphere was the private sector; she was to rear the children and occupy herself with the domestic arts. She had "her home and her housekeeping, her parish and her poultry, and all their dependent concerns."[7] Although the father was still unquestionably the head of the household, his relations with his wife and other dependents had become less authoritarian and more democratic—as we can see not only from the letters, diaries, and books of the day, but also from family portraits, where for the first time he was seated on the same plane with his wife and children. As Alexis de Tocqueville and other foreign observers noted, the American family of the 1830s was much more private than its European counterpart; it was isolated and detached from the public sphere, a haven and a refuge from the larger society.[8] It is this sentimental model of family life, with its ideal of privacy, child-centeredness, and emotional intimacy, that is still the pattern for all American families except the very poor.

Utopian experiments in family living rejected the sentimental ideal, seeing in it much that was inimical to a harmonious society. Mormon polygamy, though practiced only in ten to twenty percent of Mormon households, was an attempt to overcome the extreme individualism of American life, while the Separatists, the Shakers, and the Rappites tried, through celibacy, to elevate women to positions of equality with men. But these attempts succeeded only briefly, and only to the extent that their participants were able to isolate themselves from the larger society. As these ventures, the earlier Puritan experiment, and later the Israeli *kibbutzim* attest, utopian rearrangements of the family are usually characterized by a gradual return to the dominant norm.[9]

In the first half of the nineteenth century, the newly individualized family and the populist Jacksonian sentiment then abroad presented a joint challenge to the profession of medicine as it was taught in the medical schools of the United States and Europe. Samuel Thomson, a New Hampshire farmer who learned botanic medicine from a woman herbalist, amassed a considerable fortune when in 1806 he began to sell "Family Rights" to his practice, which was patented in 1813. For twenty dollars, customers were enrolled in his Friendly Botanic Society and received a sixteen-page booklet called *Family Botanic Medicine.* The recipes found in the booklet possessed a curious feature: they lacked mention of certain key ingredients, which the Thomsonian agent divulged only after the purchaser pledged himself never to reveal them. The agents fanned out from New England through the southern and western United States, preaching the gospel of Each Family Its Own Physician; by 1840 perhaps as many as half the citizens from Ohio to Mississippi were converts to Thomsonianism.[10]

Thomson had no use for trained physicians and refused to establish any medical schools along Thomsonian lines. In this he differed from Samuel Hahnemann, a German physician who had grown dissatisfied with the heroic therapies of professional medicine and constructed an alternate system—homeopathy—based on two laws. The first law was that to cure a disease one must give a medicine producing in healthy persons symptoms similar to those of the disease. If a compound was known to elevate a healthy pulse, for example, it could be given to someone suffering from a fever. The second law was that drugs were efficacious in inverse proportion to their amount, so that doses as small as a millionth of a gram might be given. The homeopath's "domestic kit," containing a case of tiny pills and guides to their use, became fixtures in American households from about 1835. These kits were sold not to supplant the physician but to assist families living in remote parts of the country; in serious cases, families were told, they must seek a qualified doctor. It was all so easy. Instead of the bleedings and purgings of the "allopaths" (as Hahnemannn called orthodox physicians), or the strict regimens of the Thomsonians, homeopaths offered pleasant little pills. As the allopathic Oliver Wendell Holmes observed, homeopathy "does not offend the palate, and so spares the nursery those scenes of single combat in which infants were wont to yield at length to the pressure of the spoon and the imminence of asphyxia."[11]

A third (but far less influential) variant of lay medicine aimed, like Thomsonianism, at emancipating families from doctors altogether. Hydropathy rejected drugs of every kind, whether botanic or mineral, focusing instead on sunshine, exercise, proper (vegetarian) diet, and above all, a large variety of water treatments. Devised in Silesia by Vincent Priessnitz, the methods were imported into America through the opening of water-cure establishments in New York City in the mid-1840s, thereby touching off a craze that lasted until the outbreak of the Civil War. As a water-cure family needed a physician only once (to teach the techniques), hydropaths confidently predicted the end of medical practice outside the home. The fad migrated to Battle Creek, Michigan, where John Harvey Kellogg took it up, wrote a number of monographs on the subject in the late nineteenth and early twentieth centuries, and invented corn flakes as a dietary accompaniment to the hydropathic regimen.[12]

The popularity of these sectarian, family-oriented varieties of medicine is easy to understand. In the first place, the orthodox medicine of doctors didn't have such a high success rate as to inspire universal confidence; indeed, the family-oriented competition played no small role in curbing the more heroic excesses of allopathic practice. Secondly, money was scarce for many in the antebellum era, and the vast majority of families were unable to afford a doctor's services. Thirdly, even where money was available, mere means couldn't assure care when there was no doctor nearby, as pioneers discovered to their sorrow in the great migrations West.

Postbellum Developments:
Working-Class Families and the Country Doctor

A revolution in agriculture gradually raised the standard of living for rural families in the late nineteenth century. Instead of living directly off the land, farm families sold an increasing amount of their crops for cash, which they could then use to invest in machinery that would increase production. Despite farmers' newfound prosperity, access to physicians was still a gamble. A family member would have to leave the work of the field or the farmyard to fetch the doctor, who might well be away from home caring for another patient. Most of the physician's days (and often nights) were spent traveling along backcountry roads, getting from one patient to another. As a consequence, the physician was able to see perhaps five patients a day. Geographic isolation also reduced the possibility of consultation with other doctors and limited the opportunity of learning from colleagues; the village practitioner was pretty much on his own. Notes one historian, "The first appendectomy many a doctor saw was the first he himself performed after this operation came into use in the late 1880s and the 1890s."[13]

It's little wonder, then, that doctors were eager to adopt technology that could breech the distances. The first rudimentary telephone exchange on record, built in 1877, connected the Capital Avenue Drugstore in Hartford, Connecticut, with twenty-one local doctors. As automobiles became more reliable, doctors were among the earliest to buy them. The growth of towns and cities permitted more doctors to see patients in their offices, which in turn meant they could see greater numbers of patients. Rather than using their time traveling from house to house, they could now use it to practice medicine. Shorter distances and reduced travel costs cut both ways: patients' relatives no longer lost a day's labor trying to reach a doctor, and the needs of the sick could be addressed more promptly.

The Twentieth Century's Rivalry of Care

By 1900, families had come to rely on professional medicine. Not only could they visit the doctor's office with some assurance that the doctor would be in, but institutionalized care had undergone a revolution as well. The earlier pesthouses that passed for hospitals—rat-infested places where solitary travelers who had no one else to care for them came to die—were transformed along hygienic lines into institutions where the sick could be cared for by professional nurses. Two wars helped bring about this transformation: the Crimean War, in which Florence Nightingale reduced the death rate among British troops from forty percent to two percent through improved hygiene, and the American Civil War, in which the Union Army, following her methods, organized and equipped a vast hospital system with results nearly as good.

The introduction in the 1870s of professional nurses, trained on a military model to discipline and obedience, was crucial to the success of the new hospitals, but so was the advent of antiseptic surgery, as advocated by

Joseph Lister. The traditional "kitchen surgery," done in the sufferer's home, became cumbersome with the introduction of ether and antisepsis, yet surgeons were reluctant to hospitalize their patients for fear of cross-infection. But because the new techniques permitted a growth in the volume of surgery that could be performed, surgeons were too busy for house calls. The compromise was the "medical boarding house," which provided operating facilities and acute-care nursing. This interim phase didn't last long, however. The refurbished and professionally staffed hospitals soon lost their stigma, and physicians themselves became the guiding forces for building new, smaller ones in the towns that lacked them. By 1900 surgery had become a hospital procedure.

Some physicians distrusted families who put their sick in hospitals. In an early expression of the tension between the two systems of care, Dr. W. Gill Wylie wrote in 1876 that hospitals "tend to weaken the family tie by separating the sick from their homes and their relatives, who are often too ready to relieve themselves of the burden of the sick."[14] What Wylie seems not to have noticed was the economic shift that forced urban families to depend on others for care. In the days of cottage industries, women working at home could nurse the sick in their own beds, but this care was impossible when the workplace was a factory, someone else's home, or an office. Further, as an observer pointed out in 1913, there were new space-constraints in city living. "Fewer families occupy a single dwelling, and the tiny flat or contracted apartment no longer is sufficient to accommodate sick members of the family. . . . The sick are better cared for [in hospitals] with less waste of energy, and their presence in the home does not interrupt the occupations and exhaust the means of wage earners. . . . The day of the general home care of the sick can never return."[15]

Hospitals were now more than ever places where medical science could develop, and where physicians could specialize. The attractiveness of hospital privileges was therefore an incentive for physicians to cooperate and collaborate. The sectarians, sharing most of the fundamentals of medical science with the rest of the profession, suddenly had a number of good reasons to bury their differences and work for consensus. Not only were hospital privileges worth having, but it had become logistically practical to rely on one's colleagues for referral, and for a common defense against malpractice suits. And so the family orientation of sectarian medicine gave way to a professional orientation, and medicine shifted to a corporate consciousness. This in itself would not have been enough to consolidate the profession, but it was accompanied by increased political power: licensure screened out the charlatans and the ill-educated, and the county medical societies became gatekeepers to the profession's privileges. These developments, followed by badly needed reform in the medical schools, provided the fundamental structures of organized, corporate medicine as it is practiced today.

Medicine's new power permitted it to extend its authority to commercial ventures having to do with health, and thus indirectly impinged further on family autonomy. Not only did the American Medical Association take an active role in tightening up on fraudulent proprietary drugs, it also stepped in when the Nestlè company introduced infant food. Nestlè's advertising, originally pitched to mothers ("just add water"), was by 1924 aimed at doctors; an advertisement in the *Journal of the American Medical Association* proclaimed a new product for sale "only on the prescription or recommendation of a physician. No feeding instructions appear on the trade package."[16]

The authority of medicine was also extended to public health in a broader sense. Initially a function of state and local boards of health, the goal of public health was to prevent the spread of diseases. The boards typically proceeded by quarantine, checking immigrants for symptoms of illness, teaching mothers how to care for their babies, establishing clinics for the poor, and promoting the hygiene that was seen as essential to good health. The federal government's contribution to this movement was the Public Health Service, established on military lines in 1902 as a corps of physician-officers conducting a war on such diseases as tuberculosis, bubonic plague, yellow fever, typhoid fever, and pellagra. The service's "microbe hunters" were particularly concerned to understand the disease mechanism, so that with vaccination, proper hygiene, or adequate diet the disease could be controlled. As the nation became increasingly aware of the importance of science to this quest, the government lent its support to scientific research—not basic research, as Congress was careful to specify when it established the National Institutes of Health in 1930—but research "in the problems of the diseases of man."[17]

German pharmaceutical houses led the way in synthesizing drugs from coal-tar products from about 1880, when the Friedrich Bayer Company launched sulphanol and phenacitin; the company patented a method for mass-producing aspirin a decade later. Other German chemists, working with the coal-tar derivative barbituric acid, soon synthesized Veronal and phenobarbitol. When Congress suspended all German patents during the First World War, U.S. companies began to copy the drugs, using bulk chemicals that could be bought very cheaply. Thus freed from competition, the U.S. pharmaceutical industry grew rapidly, nourished by equal parts of aggressive marketing and solid research. Perhaps even more crucial to the efforts of the drug companies was academic research, which produced (among other major discoveries) such milestones as insulin (1922), sulfa drugs (1935), and penicillin (1941–43). Better anesthesia and aseptic techniques permitted significant advances in surgery as well.

Organized medicine—professionalized, well educated, undergirded by good science and by an economic structure that allowed it to profit—was achieving unprecedented results. It could now do for the family what the family could not do for itself, and in consequence it commanded unprecedented respect. Not since the heyday of the clergy in colonial times had any profession enjoyed such trust and prestige. Physicians, too, had had their priestly function—a current running deep in medicine since the days of Aesculapius—and now they reclaimed it. They were again a holy people, ministering to the sick and the suffering with selfless devotion, set apart from the masses by an arcane and powerful knowledge. They were, moreover, technicians of the highest sophistication, white-coated scientists skilled in the use of the instruments and flasks of the laboratory. And third, they were community leaders, public-spirited citizens—kindly, decent men (and a handful of women) with the interests of society at heart.[18] In this last role lay the seeds of trouble—serious trouble that has, in the 1990s, come home to roost. But in American medicine's golden age, lasting roughly from 1900 until 1950, doctors were accorded great trust and honor.

By contrast, at the turn of the century (and at mid-century, and at the present moment, for that matter), many experts believed the family to be in a state of crisis. The U.S. divorce rate was the highest in the world: by 1916, it hit fourteen percent in Chicago, twenty percent in Los Angeles, and twenty-five percent in San Francisco. At the same time, birth rates for socially entrenched upper- and middle-class whites had fallen so far that these families were failing to reproduce themselves, while immigrant families were matching them two babies for every one—a situation that prompted Theodore Roosevelt to remark in 1903 that the middle class was committing "race suicide." As if all that weren't bad enough, more women were pursuing college educations and working outside the home, smoking cigarettes and dancing the fox trot, engaging in premarital sex and wearing rouge. The psychologist John B. Watson predicted, "In fifty years there will be no such thing as marriage."[19]

One response to a lowered birth rate was to prohibit contraception and abortion. As early as 1873, Anthony Comstock and his followers persuaded Congress to pass legislation banning the sale of "Articles of Immoral Use," along with abortifacients and the dissemination of birth control information; by 1900, physicians had convinced state legislatures across the country of the need to encourage families of "good" stock to procreate by prohibiting the practice of abortion. Despite Comstock, middle-class women sought medical help in limiting their families. A physician in 1906 noted that there was "hardly a single middle-class family" that did not expect him to help them "prevent conception."[20] The first birth control clinic was established in 1914, and from then until 1921 Margaret Sanger's crusade was highly influential in promoting the use of contraceptive devices.

If Comstock sought to ban contraception so that the birth rate of "good" families would increase, the family planning movement was concerned (among other things) to reduce the birth rate of the poor and "unfit." Ideas of social hygiene and eugenics had the stamp of medical approval, and sterilization of the underclasses was considered a progressive and humane notion:

> It was in the United States that a relatively simple form of vasectomy was developed at a penal institution around the turn of the century. This procedure, together with a rising interest in eugenics, led, by 1920, to the enactment of laws in twenty-five states providing for compulsory sterilization of the criminally insane and other people considered genetically inferior.[21]

Thus, reproductive concerns pulled in two contradictory directions. On the one hand, advanced scientific thinking favored rational control of reproduction; on the other, allowing the middle class access to the means of reproductive control eroded solid, decent, bourgeois family values.

The First World War confirmed what intellectuals, artists, and cultural trend-setters already knew: the world had turned upside down. The butchery in the trenches at Flanders Field, Château-Thierry, and along the Marne decimated Europe's youth, and the pandemic of influenza that followed hard on the heels of Armistice Day gave Americans—late entrants into the war—their own taste of wholesale death. Established orthodoxies were no longer impervious to criticism, and values one had expected to rely on no longer seemed secure. As Yeats wrote in 1921,

> Things fall apart; the centre cannot hold.
> Mere anarchy is loosed upon the world,
> The blood-dimmed tide is loosed, and everywhere
> The ceremony of innocence is drowned.[22]

In a metaphysically shaken culture that emphasized individualism and enjoyed unprecedented affluence, it is small wonder that the ideal of marriage should be one of intense mutual pleasure and companionship. In the 1920s, this striving for deep intimacy carried the sentimental ideal to new heights. Like other upper-class fashions, "companionate marriage," as it was called, was to trickle down until in the 1950s it had been adopted by middle-class, suburban families as well.

In the first half of the twentieth century, middle-class fathers became increasingly alienated from the daily concerns of domestic life—and a fear arose that mothers' undiluted influence over their children would inflict grave and irreversible psychological harm. As these fathers commuted to work in the morning, returning only at the end of the day, they tended to suppose they had discharged their familial duty through their role as breadwinner. It was not they but their wives who were now responsible for shaping the characters of their children. Child-rearing manuals—many written by doctors—counseled mothers to keep their babies on rigid four-hour schedules, and not to pick them up between feedings, on the theory that instilling regular habits in infancy could help prevent larger social problems such as delinquency, poverty, and even class antagonism. Smother-love, warned the proponents of scientific mothering, could warp children's lives.

The collapse of the stock market on Black Monday in October of 1929 propelled America into the Great Depression, a time of hardship for many families. The Depression had its impact on medicine too, for economic hard times put pressure on the profession to allow publicly subsidized health insurance to provide access to medical care. Although insurance against loss of wages due to illness had been proposed early in the century, physician opposition and U.S. entry into World War I put those proposals to sleep. By the Thirties, however, reformers mooted the question again. By now medical costs had become a more serious matter than wage loss, largely because the costs of hospitalization had increased. The argument was no longer that insurance would increase employers' profits and workers' wages, but that it would give Americans the money to pay for their "unmet medical needs."[23] As one observer pointed out in 1934,

> In former years when the range of sickness costs was lower, and few illnesses caused high expenditures, families with middle-class income felt financial pinch due to sickness much less frequently than today. Now people who are economically secure . . . against all ordinary demands, are not secure against the costs of sickness. Thus, the economic problems of medical care now implicate not merely wage-earners but the whole population.[24]

But the American Medical Association opposed mandatory health insurance as an invasion of private medical practice. Doctors' offices were standing empty and hospital beds went unused as the Depression drove more people to lose their jobs, but the AMA exhorted its members to hold fast: "Like men ashore urging self-reliance on their drowning companions, the wealthy doctors in the AMA were asking their poorer colleagues to hold the line against health insurance."[25]

Hold it they did. The New Deal, highly responsive to organized interest groups, could build Social Security out of public pressure to provide old-age pensions and unemployment insurance, but health insurance was not in the cards. The poor who would benefit by it were not influential enough to sway the legislation, and the heavy pressure from the prestigious AMA pushed directly against it.

In 1945 Truman tried again, calling upon Congress to pass a national program assuring the right to adequate medical care. Again the AMA blocked it, mounting the most expensive public relations campaign in American history up to that time—$1.5 million—against "socialized medicine." This time it wasn't just medical conservatives but conservatism generally that stalled passage of any legislation; as anticommunist sentiment rose, national health insurance no longer stood a chance.

Instead, insurance against medical expenses belonged primarily to the well off and the well organized—those who could afford to buy it privately. Those too poor to make ends meet, for whom health insurance was originally envisioned, were precisely the people who failed to receive its protection. The price the American medical profession paid for its part in all this was a visible erosion in public esteem. The image of the physician as priest and as scientist remained intact, but his image as the community leader took a severe drubbing:

> The Socialized medicine debates undermined public confidence in medicine as a profession. The heavily financed publicity campaigns undertaken in the name of the A.M.A. generated political statements that few people could take seriously and raised questions about the claims of members of the profession acting in scientific and clinical roles. Even before World War II the evident social insensitivity of physician groups such as the A.M.A. tended to tarnish the doctor as a public figure, and many people began to associate the physician with another familiar stereotype, the small businessman, who was presumably not only grasping but slightly dishonest.[26]

People still very much wanted the services the physician could offer, and they distinguished sharply between their own family physician (whom they trusted) and "doctors" (whom they trusted a bit less). The profession as a whole, however, has never fully recovered from these struggles against universal access to care.

Contemporary Families and Medicine

The postwar period witnessed a dramatic growth in the scale of American medicine—an immense medical-research establishment and the most scientifically advanced hospitals in the world. Before World War II, over seventy-five percent of doctors described themselves as general practitioners. By 1949, the percentage calling themselves specialists had jumped to thirty-seven, and by 1966 this jumped again to sixty-nine percent. In the surgical specialties, the growth was the most dramatic: from ten percent of the profession in 1931 to over thirty percent by 1969.[27] Because medical work was concentrated in hospitals and doctors' offices, the average private physician was able, by 1950, to see one hundred patients per week—double the number seen in 1930.

If practices and specialties expanded, so did the technologies physicians could offer patients. Kidney dialysis machines, ventilators, organ transplants, CAT scans, lithotripsy, nuclear medicine—all have become widely available and routinely offered in the last two decades, albeit at a staggering cost. Americans now spend fifteen percent of the Gross Domestic Product (GDP) on health care—more than on education and defense combined—and the figure is still climbing. Many attribute the rise in expenditure to Medicare and Medicaid, inaugurated in 1965, but these only reinforced an existing problem. In hospitals, where the new and complex procedures involving sophisticated equipment and technologies were performed, "the clamor for more resources was constant, relentless, and plausible. But the cause of rising costs was not so much the intensity of the clamor as the financial arrangements that allowed hospitals to yield to it."[28] Third party payers, reimbursing providers on a fee-for-service basis, insulated patients and providers alike from the true cost of treatment decisions and so reduced the incentive to keep costs under control.

Distrust of big business and a general emphasis on individual rights prompted Americans in the 1970s to view medicine with a skeptical eye, and in the 1980s a swing toward conservatism prompted more skepticism. Tax money and government functions were returned to the private sector, thus perpetuating a lack of central planning and a patchwork system driven largely by profit motives. As government and business continue to seek control over medical costs, and as medicine continues to come to grips with its corporate persona, doctors can expect their profession to undergo even further strain.

The fair distribution of health care resources has become a political problem of major proportions, and the demographic shift toward an aging population in need of long-term (and expensive) care will not ease it. In 1995, approximately thirty-eight million people—most of them the working poor and their children—have no health insurance at all, and at least twice that number are badly underinsured. Sophisticated medical resources go mainly to those who can pay for them, while Medicaid funding becomes increasingly insufficient. Because poor families cannot afford to immunize their children, the United States in 1991 had the worst vaccination record for children under two years old of any country in the Western Hemisphere.[29] While the Clinton Administration has taken steps to improve matters, about sixty percent of two-year-olds still have not been immunized, according to a report by the Carnegie Corporation released in April 1994. The same report announced that nine in one thousand U.S. babies die before their first birthday—one of the highest infant mortality rates in the industrialized world.[30]

Despite these concerns, Americans continue to place a high premium on health care—and indeed, the furor over universal access to it makes sense only if the care is genuinely valuable. Among the top fifteen causes of death, the ten that have declined in the last two decades are the ones most responsive to medical treatment; similarly, studies of special efforts to improve prenatal, child, and maternal health show clearly that the services of doctors did make a difference.[31] Medicine prolongs life, though no one has yet determined how much credit is due to other factors, such as improved hygiene, nutrition, and pollution control. Moreover, medical care reduces disability, disfigurement, pain, and confusion about the nature of experience. America's strong faith in medicine, then, is not without warrant.

How has the American family fared in the second half of the century? U.S. entry into World War II raised people's incomes, but it also increased the cost of living. For the first time, as their husbands entered the armed forces, a large number of married women entered the workforce—accompanied by official dollops of guilt. The government sent out a strong, mixed message:

> On the one hand, women were repeatedly told by the federal government that victory could not be achieved without their entry into the labor force. On the other, the federal government declared, "Now, as in peacetime, a mother's primary duty is to her home and children."[32]

Whirlwind courtships, the pangs of separation when servicemen were shipped overseas, the pitifully small allotment checks, and shortages of everything from housing to razor blades—all this had its effect on families in wartime. Teenagers became a distinct group: zoot-suited boys roamed the streets in gangs, fighting with brass knuckles, blackjacks, and guns made out of four-inch lengths of pipe, while gangs of girls known as "wolf packs" sprang up in big cities. Adolescent prostitution was on the rise. The American public worried in a new and vocal way that absent fathers, domineering mothers, and inadequate child care would result in wholesale psychological maladjustment. Philip Wylie's *A Generation of*

Vipers, a best-seller in 1942, convinced millions that psychological immaturity was caused by paternal absenteeism and maternal dominance and overprotectiveness. Family welfare, now as never before, had become a function of mental health. In the view of many, it was high time Father came home and the family settled down.

That is precisely what, in the Fifties, it tried to do. The watchword for the family was "togetherness," and it was to be practiced in the suburbs, where low mortgage interest rates and cheap fuel for the family car put middle-class life in easy reach. The division of labor was once again drawn along gender lines: married women were to leave their wartime offices and factories, and men were to reoccupy them. Marriage was seen as central to a happy and meaningful life, and woman's place was in the home, looking after the children. Television and the popular literature of the decade reinforced this *Father Knows Best* ideal, and so did politicians. In 1955, Adlai E. Stevenson told the women graduating from Smith College that their task was to "restore valid, meaningful purpose to life in your home," and to keep their husbands "truly purposeful." "Influence us, man and boy," he exhorted.[33] This image of family life, with the father as primary breadwinner and the mother as primary caregiver, and all centered affectionately around the children, still has its grip on the collective American imagination.

The suburbs ran the spectrum from exclusive, tree-lined neighborhoods to Levittown's dense rows of assembly-line tract houses, to ethnically divided working-class neighborhoods. What they all had in common, however, was a high turnover rate. In the suburbs around the city of New York, fewer than six percent of people climbing the corporate ladder were still living in the same house in 1960 as in 1955. Relocation and the relative isolation of women and children put increased pressure on the family to meet its members' emotional needs. Spouses looked to each other not only for love, but for the companionship and moral support that in more settled times had been provided by friends and extended kin. The companionate ideal of marriage developed by the well-to-do in the 1920s—itself an intensification of the two-centuries-old sentimental model—now became the model for the middle class.

But the dream of "togetherness" had, after all, been unrealistic. After a dip attributable to war-weariness, the divorce rate continued to rise by the steady three percent per decade that had characterized it since the Civil War. Women were torn by the desire to be good mothers and by the call to fulfillment outside the home. The birth control pill, introduced in 1960, offered new reliability in family planning, but it was also a way in which medicine increased women's independence from the family altogether. The Civil Rights movement in the deep South and in northern cities, couched in the language of liberation, sounded a cry to freedom that was echoed by college students resistant to creeping U.S. involvement in Viet Nam. Sexual revolution, experimentation with recreational drugs, and general rebelliousness against established values became the marks of a youth culture that romanticized individual, subjective experience.

The cry of freedom was then taken up by women, who left kitchen and carpools in increasing numbers to become breadwinners. The proportion of working women with preschoolers jumped from twelve percent in 1950 to forty-five percent in 1980, and women with older children joined the workforce in even greater numbers. By 1994, more than half the mothers of infants worked outside the home.[34] The divorce rate continued to rise: in 1979 and 1981 it was 5.3 per thousand (per year, among all married couples), producing projections that fifty percent of recent marriages would end in divorce. This figure fluctuated and declined in the 1980s, and from 1988 on the rate has been a steady 4.7 per thousand, which works out to a 48.4 percent chance that the marriage will not last.[35]

"No-fault" divorce laws have been economically hard on women. Many studies have shown that men's economic status improves after divorce, while women's and children's worsens considerably. When in 1970 California became the first state to adopt the "no-fault" approach, the financial discrepancy increased. In 1960, the per capita income of divorced women was already a mere sixty-two percent of the income of divorced men, but by 1980 the gap had widened to fifty-six percent. In fact, in the first year after divorce, the average standard of living for men rose by forty-two percent, while that of women fell by seventy-three percent. The explanation is that "no-fault" laws assume economic equality between men and women both within marriage and in the society at large, but the assumption is false.

> Divorcing men and women are not, of course, equal, both because the
> two sexes are not treated equally in society and, as we have seen, because

typical, gender-structured marriage makes women socially and economically vulnerable. The treatment of unequals as if they were equals has
long been recognized as an obvious instance of injustice.[36]

Twenty-five percent of all dependent children now live with only one
parent, and in ninety percent of cases, that parent is their mother.[37] The
vast majority of women rearing children on their own are divorced or separated; only a small percentage have never been married. Yet for the very
poor, welfare regulations actually discourage marriage. As the law presently stands, if a mother receiving Aid to Families with Dependent Children
money marries, the stepfather must support the children and AFDC payments stop. Further, in twenty-nine states, the presence of the father in the
household, even if he is unemployed, automatically renders his family
ineligible for AFDC payments. To assure that his wife and children receive
assistance, he must desert them.

If, then, primarily through divorce but also through desertion the
majority of poor families are headed by women, it is also true that these
women receive support and help from a network of kin and neighbors. In
urban ghettos those suffering the worst poverty—whether Mexican
Americans, black Hispanics, African Americans, or those of other ethnic
backgrounds—tend to form webs of kith and kin that serve as the basic
unit of social organization. While extreme poverty can be an inheritance
that is passed on to subsequent generations, few families headed by single
women remain poor for very long. Most have recently experienced divorce
or separation, and most leave the welfare rolls within two years.[38]

Family-related problems continue to grow. The number of children
who live in poverty as a result of divorce, though leveling off, is a matter of
grave concern. A related but distinct set of problems has to do with the
family's response to working mothers of young children: affordable day
care is in seriously short supply, fathers are only slowly coming to see the
need to share domestic labor, and the job market is ill-equipped to accommodate familial needs.[39] Further, the problem of violence against women
continues to plague families. The Bureau of Justice Statistics of the U.S.
Department of Justice reports that between 1979 and 1987, women were
victims of violent intimates at a rate three times that of men—6.3 per
thousand compared to 1.8 per thousand. Over the nine-year period,
women reported 10.2 million violent attacks by strangers and 5.6 million

attacks by intimates, 1.9 million of which were committed by ex-spouses and 1.7 million of which were committed by boyfriends. The average annual number of victimizations was 625,800. Eighty-five percent of these crimes were assaults, three percent were rapes, and for one woman in five the crime was one in a series of at least three similar assaults sustained within the previous six months.[40] And these figures are conservative. Testimony to the U.S. Senate in 1991 estimated that there are as many as four million incidents of domestic violence against women each year—a figure six times greater than the Department of Justice statistics.[41]

Notwithstanding the problems, however, families continue to form. Three-fourths of divorced women and five-sixths of divorced men—eighty percent of whom have minor children—remarry, and the second marriage generally holds.[42] Despite experiments at intimate living without benefit of court or clergy, most people get married in their mid-twenties—as they have for centuries. Gay and lesbian couples receive increased media attention as they attempt to form long-term, socially recognized families that frequently involve bearing or adopting children. Orphan asylums are extinct, partly because there are fewer orphans but partly also because the orphans who remain have been placed in foster care, so they can enjoy the good things of family life. It seems, then, that recurrent reports of the family's death have greatly been exaggerated.

Morals of the Story

What are we to make of all this? If a quick look at the history of the American family and American medicine shows us nothing else, it reveals that stress, turmoil, and identity crises are nothing new for either institution. Other themes endure as well. Despite recurrent crises, despite shifts in ideology and economics, both medicine and families have attempted to address very basic forms of human vulnerability. They are a bulwark against illness, suffering, and death; they respond to our need to bear and nurture children, to live in intimacy with others, to form the future. But against this backdrop of endurance, a drama of immense change is playing itself out. Medicine may have lost a substantial amount of the charismatic power it once wielded—it is harder these days to take seriously the image of physician as priest—but it has acquired unprecedented economic, technological, and social power, none of which it fully understands how to direct or to share. The family, for its part, pretty much adheres to the sentimental (and somewhat internally unstable) form it took on over two centuries ago—modified in middle-class families by women's increasing labor outside the home.

Medicine's power and the corporate model through which it expresses that power have had their impact on the relationship between doctor and patient. As medicine underwent its corporate transformation, doctors increasingly abandoned the assumption that they knew what was best for their patients and moved to a heightened scrupulousness about respecting their patients' right to self-determination. This shift was fueled by the bioethics movement, which, in showing physicians that the values that supported their practice were not all medical ones, has for the last twenty-five years emphasized the importance of seeing patients as individuals whose preferences must be honored. As twentieth-century American corporate life is geared toward individual consumer preference in any case, the new bioethical orientation has not been so terribly difficult for the transformed medical profession to assimilate. Medicine, whose ethics has always been patient-centered, became even more so. The most significant change is that it is often patients, at the center of medical practice, and not just their physicians, who determine what is in their medical interests.

This development continues to be much celebrated, despite economic pressures to start counting costs as well as patient preference. But should we as a society be promoting a practice of medicine whose moral center is the will of the individual patient? This individualism, now so exaggerated that doctors (and even some ethicists) are suspicious of a patient who exhibits concern for others, has joined forces with other values growing out of medical science (including both a heavy reliance on ever-more-sophisticated technology and a denial of death) to magnify the difference between the code of the physician and the values of the family, thereby causing unnecessary suffering for families and physicians alike.

Understanding the tensions between these two systems of ethics is the task of this book. As a story is worth a thousand explanations, we offer two, both troubling, to illustrate the kinds of conflict we have in mind.

CARING FOR TONY

Tony, who is twenty-four years old, has been hospitalized about a hundred times in the course of his life. He is small and thin, with the voice and body of a boy half his age, but with an IQ of 142 and an excellent record as a full-time graduate student in the fine arts. Afflicted by an unusual form of muscular dystrophy, he has outlived his life expectancy by about six years. He is very proud of each year, seeing his survival as a contribution to medical knowledge that may someday help others who suffer from his disease.

When he was diagnosed, Tony's parents were told he would not live to adulthood, and he became the center of the family's life. So that they could devote themselves to Tony, his parents often sent his sisters, Angela and Rosalie, to stay with relatives; they blamed each other for causing his illness. Family life revolved around the "dying child."

When Tony was eight and Angela sixteen she married to escape her brother-centered family, but five years later it was Angela who nursed her father as he lay dying of a stroke, and then her mother, who after two more years died of breast cancer. Her mother's last words were, "Take care of your brother." Angela and her husband have done their best, taking him into their own home to live with their two chldren. Except for educational scholarships and for Medicaid, which pays for his enormous medical bills, Angela and her husband have supported Tony financially and emotionally.

Tony is finishing up a stint in a rehabilitation hospital that is teaching him to be more independent in caring for himself; he'll be ready for discharge in about a month. He has been actively involved in his program and ought to be fairly independent when he leaves the hospital. He has not made friends, although he seems to like his occupational therapist and is teaching her how to draw. When he is discharged he plans to return to Angela's home so that she and her family can continue to look after him.

Angela has been having thoughts of suicide. She cries all the time and is constantly tired. Tony demands a lot of attention, so Angela's day, beginning at 5:30 AM and ending at 11:00 PM, is spent cooking, cleaning, and taking care of Tony. Both teenage children resent him; her husband "has had it." He tells Tony's social worker that Tony is a spoiled brat whose demands on the family are destroying it. When Tony is discharged, neither Angela nor her husband wants him back in their home.

Tony's other sister, Rosalie, is now twenty-eight. She too is married and has three children. She's aware of what Angela is going through and refuses to help in any way. In her view, Tony ruined her childhood, killed her parents, and is now killing her sister. She has explained this to Tony's social worker, declaring, "I'm not gonna let him get me too!"

The social worker is certainly sympathetic to both sisters, but she is worried about Tony's right to self-determination, and his right to care. He *is* dying, after all, and he ought not to die among strangers. The whole point of rehabilitation has been to make him as physically autonomous as possible; his moral autonomy must be respected as well.[43]

DECIDING FOR CHRIS

When Chris Busalacchi was two years old, her mother died, leaving her and her sister Jill in the care of their father. Pete Busalacchi, grieving for his wife, cast a shadow of sorrow over his daughters' childhood. Their upbringing was not always smooth; sometimes there were angry quarrels. But his conversations with them typically ended with, "That's my girl," and the girls would respond, "That's my dad." It was an uneasy sign of affection.

In 1987, when Chris was seventeen, she was badly injured in a car accident. Her left arm and leg were broken, but worse were the head injuries that elevated her intracranial pressure to five times the normal level. She lay in a persistent vegetative state in a rehabilitation center in St. Louis, Missouri, her upper brain so severely damaged that she would never again be able to speak, think, or feel any kind of pain. Her brain stem was still functional, causing her to chew constantly and gag frequently on her saliva. Her right leg was bent so that her knee was always in the air.

Her father wanted Chris's feeding tube withdrawn so that her body could die. "All of us who love her would like to see her body finally at peace," he said in 1990, after a three-year struggle with the health-care center and the courts. "The automobile accident took the real Chris from us a long time ago." But that year the Supreme Court held that the state of Missouri can insist on "clear and convincing" evidence that a now-incapacitated patient would have refused medical treatment. In the absence of "clear" proof that Chris herself would have wanted the feeding tube removed, the State has the power to decide the tube must stay.

Her father remained convinced—as was the Missouri judge—that no one would wish this "life" on one's worst enemy. "I made many a decision to guide her into adulthood," lamented Pete Busalacchi, "and now, when she's incapable of deciding for herself, the state wants to take the place of her father." In December 1990, he attempted to move his daughter to Minnesota, where families are allowed more discretion in cases of this kind. This touched off a series of legal maneuvers on the part of the State of Missouri that finally came to an end in January 1993, when a new state attorney general, who had campaigned on the promise to end Missouri's involvement in the case, was sworn in. His move to dismiss the most recent appeal to the state supreme court was granted, and in late February the feeding tube was removed. Chris died on 7 March 1993, six years after her family first began to mourn her loss.[44]

In the stories of Tony and Chris we can see some of the friction between two systems of care. In both cases, medical caregivers conscientiously and successfuly practiced their profession according to the dictates and privileges that have accrued to it over the course of the last two centuries. They employed not only a large range of technologies but also empathy and compassion for the patient. In both cases, their doing so led to hardship for the families that no one—least of all the physicians and other caregivers—intended. In Tony's case, the family was asked to provide amounts of care that threatened to sink it completely. In Chris's case, her family was barred from making what many would regard as a reasonable decision on her behalf, even though its members had remained closely involved in her care. Here the family was deprived of a prerogative that families in earlier times would have held without question. The uneasy tensions at the center of these two stories are repeated over and over in other people's lives, and it is not likely that they will go away of their own accord. They must be examined, carefully described, and thoughtfully debated if we are to achieve any kind of public consensus about the way families and medicine can be helped to greater harmony as they tend to the needs of the sick.

Chapter Two

Why Families Matter

EVERYBODY KNOWS WHAT A FAMILY IS. Even if the ones we grew up in don't much resemble our favorite image, we nonetheless feel strongly that the family:

- is perfectly exemplified by the Jacksons. Joe Jackson works for an electronics firm. He puts in long hours, but his wife Judy is at home with their two children, Julie and Jeff, who are both in elementary school. The Jacksons live in a suburb of their town and own their own home. Both sets of grandparents live within easy driving distance, and at Thanksgiving and Christmas the aunts and uncles and cousins gather at the Jacksons' house for wonderful family reunions;

—or—

- is perfectly exemplified by the Garcias. Pedro and Consuela Garcia and their four children and all the in-laws and extended family live within a four-block radius in the Texas town where they have lived for generations; Pedro's uncle is the present patriarch of the clan. The Garcias are devoted to each other and would do anything to help a member of the family;

—or—

- is perfectly exemplified by the Tuggles. Marge has two daughters, twelve and fourteen, by a former marriage, and is having problems with her present husband, Tom. They have violent quarrels over money, especially when they've been drinking, and Tom sometimes beats Marge as well as the girls. The fourteen-year-old has been sexually abused by her stepfather; the twelve-year-old has run away from home;

—or—

- is perfectly exemplified by Zach Tyson. His drug-addicted mother abandoned him when he was an infant; she herself didn't know who his father was. He grew up in a series of foster homes with no one in particular to care about him, so that by the age of eleven he was an alcoholic who brought gin to school every day in a cardboard milk carton. He's the poster boy for the new age, in which the family has become so seriously dysfunctional it is close to worthless.

—or—

- is exemplified by some lively, if not logically impeccable, mixture of these themes of kinship, affection, conflict, and exhaustion.

Often we resolve conflicting images of the family by attributing positive images to the past and negative ones to the present. Nor are we the first generation to do so; the fall of the family from a past golden age is a theme as old as Genesis, sounded again in Virgil's *Georgics* and Shakespeare's *King Lear,* reechoed by Edmund Burke and Edward Gibbon. But as the sociologist William J. Goode points out,

> a single individual is not likely to be an excellent observer of an entire society, or the whole family system, because he or she has not had much opportunity to observe those other families first hand. It is even more difficult for individuals to be accurate about time trends that extend beyond one person's lifetime. This difficulty creates perhaps the commonest error in attempting to chart family changes. It is an error that is self-contradictory: the commentator asserts that in his lifetime family patterns are changing rapidly, but that in some relatively recent past (usually his grandfather's time) family patterns were much more stable, for they followed the ancient and rightful ways of old. Since people are likely to have made such remarks in almost every generation, clearly they cannot all be correct.[1]

Just as clearly, some *could* be correct. It certainly seems as if the contemporary family is changing for the worse. Given that recent marriages have only a 48.4 percent chance of avoiding divorce, given the incidence of child abuse, teenage pregnancy, and drug addiction beginning as early as the fourth grade, given the prevalence of domestic violence, given the major scars parents inflict on their children's psyches even when they love them and want to do well by them, why should we care that medicine is exerting pressure that threatens to erode families even further?[2] Why not let them die a natural death?

Certain social critics, on the left in particular, have been quick to call for the abolition of the family, because it has the unpleasant habit of passing on to new generations old patterns of injustice and oppression.[3] Even the liberal thinker John Rawls, widely regarded as today's most influential political philosopher, has suggested that the family may be a barrier to the achievement of a just state. Rawls points out that family circumstances greatly affect children's ability to cultivate their native talents. Besides, families have the power to develop or not develop in their children such dispositions as industry and determination, which are necessary for social success. Given these facts, Rawls concludes, "The principle of fair equality of opportunity can only be imperfectly carried out, at least as long as the institution of the family exists."[4]

Critics on the right, like those on the left, tend to think families have taken a turn for the worse, but rather than scrap them outright they call for a return to more traditional values that will allow them "once again" to become the havens of domestic comfort and the cradles of morality they used to be.[5] The conservative ideal looks suspiciously like the middle-class ideal of the 1950s: the division of labor follows strict gender lines; the home not only contains children but is child-centered; women and children in particular (but to some extent men also) submerge their individuality to the common domestic good.

But the ideal is both older and deeper than nostalgia for a *Leave It to Beaver* past; in his *Enquiry Concerning the Principles of Morals* (1777), David Hume noted how affection within families can dissolve individual difference, or, to vary the metaphor, "Between married persons, the cement of friendship is by the laws supposed so strong as to abolish all division of possessions; and has often, in reality, the force ascribed to it."[6]

Building on this notion, the contemporary political philosopher Michael Sandel has invented an interesting response to those who condemn the family as unjust: he argues that, at least in those intimate relationships where "generosity of spirit" prevails, justice shouldn't matter very much.[7]

Views of the Family: Romantic, Cynical, or Confused

Conservative images of the family are romantic, at once idealistic and intimate, and they place great emphasis on the merged identities of intimacy. Spouses are—in a strong sense of the metaphor—one flesh, shared selves, and their children carry the parental identities into the future in a kind of immortality. There seems little room here for gay or lesbian families, for childless couples, for open marriages, or for children in joint physical custody.

If this strongly communitarian view of the family is romantic, its negation is cynical. It is cynical because it is disillusioned, having tacitly assumed the romantic view and then discovered that we fall far short of this ideal. Understanding the potential for tyranny and slavery when individuals become fused, the cynic settles for individuation and separation, assuming competing interests among family members and distrusting the possibility of altruism. This is of course a caricature, but in its subtler manifestations it underlies many of the contemporary critiques of families.

It seems to us that both romanticism and cynicism must be avoided if we are to come to any kind of sensible understanding of the problem that has arisen between families and medicine. The romantic and the cynic each see something that is true about families, but neither perspective permits them to flourish. It is the business of families to maintain a continued tension between the fusion of the one and the individuation of the other. If the tension isn't present, the family disintegrates: either it collapses under unrealistic demands for emotional fulfillment, or its members drift off to pursue their personal projects in splendid isolation.

We might also note a third view of the family that has recently come into fashion—the family as "dissolved" by too many conflicting configurations. Consider Fred Rosner's contradictory use of the term in the following passage:

> Unfortunately, in 1991 the family is no longer perceived as the backbone of civilized humanity. Many children grow up in one-parent families

because of the high divorce rate. Many couples do not marry but simply live together. Many single people remain that way. Some homosexuals and lesbians are trying to create a new definition of family. Some one-parent families result, not from divorce, but from abandonment by one of the parents. Some single women have children by insemination of donor sperm. Surrogate women bear children for others, including homosexuals and transsexuals.[8]

The argument these observations are intended to support is that it's no use trying to sort out a physician's relationship with the patient's family because often there *is* no family in the sense that Rosner understands it.

The trouble may be that Rosner is assuming there is some defining essence of "family" that is not present in the above-mentioned configurations. But this is a difficulty that can be overcome by letting go of the idea that families *have* a defining essence. Instead, we can think of families as people clustered into configurations that have at least some of a rather wide array of characteristics, no one of which is definitive, but most of which will be present to one degree or another. Particular families will possess many of these characteristics; we can note what the philosopher Ludwig Wittgenstein called "family resemblances" among them. Characteristics common to most families, for example, are adult relationships of emotional, economic, and sexual intimacy, often marked by vows of fidelity and commitment to the long term; relationships of blood kinship; relationships marked by shared histories born of close and ongoing contact. These relationships are part of what we mean by "family" in the sense of household: "an aggregate or group of actual (living) members, who are closely associated by living arrangement or by commitment, for better or worse." This sense of "family" can be distinguished from a second sense—that of the family in the abstract: "an idea or an ideal that refers to a family name or genetic line, the extended family in the largest sense, whose boundaries or members extend over both space and time."[9] We are concerned with both senses of the word as we try to relieve the friction between family and medicine.

What Families Are Good for: Making Selves

If we are to think carefully about the charge that families (using the word in the "household" sense) have become dysfunctional—if, that is, we consider what truth there is in the cynic's view—we must begin by identifying the more important functions families ordinarily perform. Reproduction for the most part takes place within families and is accompanied by other functions that Sara Ruddick has identified as the tasks of maternal work: preserving the child from harm, nurturing the child, and socializing the child.[10] In all families, with or without children, the same three tasks are performed for mature members as well—our vulnerabilities are protected, everyone is fed, clothed, and sheltered, and familial pressure is exerted to encourage individuals to adjust to the larger society. While these functions are all in principle separable from one another, they are in fact not separated in almost any known family system.[11]

Perhaps even more valuable than the protecting, nurturing, and socializing functions of families is their central importance to human identity—they play the primary role in making us the people we are. The family therapist Salvador Minuchin puts it this way:

> In all cultures, the family imprints its members with selfhood. Human experience of identity has two elements: a sense of belonging and a sense of being separate. The laboratory in which these ingredients are mixed and dispensed is the family, the matrix of identity.
>
> In the early process of socialization, families mold and program the child's behavior and sense of identity. The sense of belonging comes with an accommodation on the child's part to the family groups and with his assumption of transactional patterns in the family structure that are consistent throughout different life events. Tommy Wagner is a Wagner, and throughout his life he will be the son of Emily and Mark. This will be an important factor in his existence. . . . Every member's sense of identity is influenced by his sense of belonging to a specific family.
>
> The sense of separateness and individuation occurs through participation in different family subsystems in different family contexts, as well as through participation in extrafamilial groups. As the child and the family grow together, the accommodation of the family to the child's needs delimits areas of autonomy that he experiences as separateness. A psychological and transactional territory is carved out for that particular child. Being Tom is different from being a Wagner.[12]

Tommy's self is forged through his relationships to other family members, in the intimacy characteristic of family life. When we live in close and affectionate proximity with others, we can be seen and celebrated specially; we can be known more fully than our relationships in the workplace, in civic life, or in casual friendships permit. Being known well—being seen lovingly and particularly, in a way that singles us out from the billions of others who walk in the world—reinforces our understanding of who we are. As our intimates respond to what they come to know of us, we turn their response into a fuller knowledge of ourselves. By the same token, if we are not seen lovingly, we learn to accept whatever negative image of ourselves our family happens to offer; especially when we are children, but also when we are grown, those with whom we live in intimacy have a terrible power over us.

Can we have selves if we don't have families? Of course. The culture we inhabit, the language we speak, the practices and customs of our society, even when conveyed to us through the nonintimates we encounter in childhood, are important sources of personal identity. The question is one of scale. The unit of the family permits each member to be seen more particularly and specially than is possible, say, in an orphanage or boarding school, and there is an intensity to the relationship that, for good or ill, leaves its mark more deeply than the impersonal relationships formed in early life.

Using Power to Make Selves

The power of parents over their children is the most terrible, because it is easiest to misuse. One such misuse occurs when parents fail to acknowledge their power—when, for example, they fail to set limits for the child out of a misplaced regard for the child's autonomy, or when they become psychologically fused to the child in ways that invite sexual abuse. In other families, power is acknowledged but is used to hurt or belittle the child rather than serving the child's welfare; when power is used in this way the child is tyrannized. The third misuse of power occurs when parents refuse to share it with their children, when the T-shirt slogan, "Because I'm the daddy, that's why," becomes emblematic of how the child is denied appropriate participation in its exercise.

When parental power is systematically misused, children bear the mark of it all their lives. No one knows the precise extent of child abuse in the U.S.; like rape, it is probably underreported, and, also like rape, it is difficult to clearly define. A 1994 study reports that one in three victims of physical abuse is a child.[13] The *Journal of the American Medical Association* recently reported that the annual serious injury rate to children of nondrinking mothers was 4.5 percent, while for children of mothers who were problem drinkers the rate was ten percent.[14] A California study, which was reported in the same issue of the journal, defines as "abuse" everything from a mild slap to violent kicking and choking; in that study, forty-two percent of the 1025 college students surveyed reported that their fathers physically assaulted them as adolescents, and forty-nine percent said their mothers assaulted them. "Mothers tended to use the milder forms of violence, such as slapping. Fathers kicked, punched, choked, and beat up their children more often than did the mothers."[15]

If the broad definition of abuse in this study points up the problem of generating reliable data on the prevalence of physical abuse of children, sexual touching of children by their parents ought arguably always to count as abuse. It can, however, be terribly difficult to determine that such touching has actually taken place. Clinical studies have suggested that girls are sexually abused seven to nine times more often than boys, although more comprehensive, nonclinical studies reduce the ratio to two to one. In one study of male and female college students who suffered long-term abuse as children, forty-four percent of their abusers were family members.[16] A sexually abusive father or stepfather (or, far less frequently, a mother) can inflict particularly grievous harm to the child's sense of self, because children depend on their parents for information about how the world fits together and what counts as normal behavior—both of which are grossly distorted when a child is molested. To compound the harm, an eroticized child may also be a willing participant. Her predator may be able to coopt the child into consenting, enjoying, cooperating—and so corrupt as well as enslave her:

> If she balks at doing what he wants, he takes it out on her and the rest of the family. He treats the girl as the tyrannized wife, a beleaguered peacemaker. He gets angry and lashes out at others but blames her, and she believes him. If she plays his games, he will pay her. The pay locks her in still further, since she now sees herself as consenting and therefore corrupt, cooperating with her corrupt father. Thus, step by step he leads an eight-year-old into playing, at one and the same time, the roles of the self-sacrificing wife and the whore.
>
> Incest violates the child at the deepest possible levels—by bruising not the body but the inner sanctum, the child's very identity. She senses her self not confidently, as loved, but as exploited, eroticized. An identity, still obscure to the self, makes itself felt now, not in the urgency of love but in a "sick, twisty, horrible feeling."
>
> Suffering twists and wrenches the core self out of shape or splits it in two.[17]

Yet the same power that can shatter the child's self is also the power that can forge that self. When it is used properly, parents *own* their power: they accept responsibility for wielding it and shield their children from its uncontrolled destruction. They also *aim* their power to appropriate ends: they use it to do the maternal work that must be done for the child, and not to get the pleasure of controlling others. And third, they *share* their power: they gradually give more and more of it to the child as the child becomes old enough to set and achieve her own goals. The physician-philosopher Howard Brody has offered this analysis of owning, aiming, and sharing for understanding the power doctors have over patients;[18] as it fits any relationship in which there is a legitimate imbalance of power, we adopt it here for families.

If the family properly uses its power to "imprint its members with self-hood," its children will achieve both a sense of belonging and a sense of separateness. They will become neither romantically fused with others in the family, nor cynically free-floating. But how do families accomplish this? By sharing *themselves* with the child, they bring him to feel he belongs to the family; by sharing *their power* with the child, they allow him to become himself, different from the rest of the family.

In a process of continued interaction, parents, stepparents, siblings, grandparents share themselves with the child, who is drawn by need and by affection to adopt their values, mannerisms, tastes, and dispositions as its own. The family shares its categories of meaning with the child, and it shares the family stories (often told by grandmothers) that give children their sense of place among the family's generations. In these ways, children acquire the most deeply satisfying version of their own particular, ongoing place in the world. They achieve their sense of belonging.

The sense of separateness is achieved through shared power. As family members stand back and allow children to use their own judgment, children come to a more prudent exercise of such judgment. Empowered to participate in various familial subsystems, and encouraged to form relationships outside the family, children gain an understanding that it is right and good to be different from others. When this difference is achieved through shared power rather than through scapegoating or other destructive forms of isolation, children gain what is perhaps the most valuable good of all—their self-respect.

Teaching Children to Be Good

At the same time as they impart the sense of sameness and the sense of separateness, families impart in their children a sense of the reality of other persons that is the foundation of morality. We begin life with no ego boundaries, unable to distinguish between ourselves and the world around us. When we learn self-respect—that is, when we come to understand and honor our own distinctiveness within the safe setting of the love of others—we also begin to learn about the distinctiveness of other people. It is our families who take us on the journey from egoism to intimacy to sociability. As they do, we come to recognize first that those we love must be treated with care and respect, and, later, that strangers also require such treatment. Through our acquaintance with the particular projects, idiosyncrasies, temperaments, and desires of those with whom we live in intimacy, we come to take seriously the personhood of others, and the moral stance such personhood implies.

If a sense of the reality of other persons is the foundation of morality, a "thick" conception of the morally good life, shared with others, is the foundation of community. By "thick" we mean a richly detailed vision of life that most or all members of a group hold in common. A Benedictine abbey is a good example of such a conception—the monks share not only an ancient tradition and a common understanding of how to live out one's religious beliefs, but are bound together by certain vows and common practices that reflect important values they share as a community. Families have the potential for offering their children a miniature community that is equally—though differently—"thick." Families might, of course, simply mirror the interest-group liberalism characteristic of late twentieth-century American public life—a system in which everyone is afforded maximum liberty to pursue his or her own interests, defined "thinly" in whatever way the person chooses, providing no one else is hurt in the pursuit. But as the philosopher Laura Purdy has pointed out, the assumptions of rights and freedom underlying the liberal state rest on a domestic morality that is not self-interested at all, but rather directed toward the good of others. "The public realm works only if many real human needs are taken care of somewhere else—a place where the individualistic conception of human relations predicated of that realm do not hold."[19] That place has typically been the family, whose morality is not individualistic but communal, and whose members do what has been aptly referred to as the "shadow-work" of caring for those who are too young, frail, or ill to be out in the public realm pursuing their own interests. The liberal state cannot function without this shadow-work.

There is some evidence, however, that families are abandoning their communal view of the good life and embracing the current libertarian assumptions of the public sphere. In 1983 the popular sociologist Vance Packard cited a Yankelovich study of the American family reporting that forty-three percent of "new breed" parents put self-fulfillment and duty to self above duty to others, even their own children. The attitude seemed to be, "I want to be free, so why shouldn't you children be free? We will not sacrifice for you because we have our own life to lead. But when you are grown, you owe us nothing." These parents were unwilling to act in ways that would instill more sociable attitudes in their children, nor did they teach such values.[20] If a shift of this kind is indeed taking place within families, the implications are most disturbing, not only for children and the infirm, but for the liberal state as a whole. Somehow, the needs of those who do not fit the model of the rational, autonomous self-asserter must be met; somewhere, we all must satisfy those needs that are not for rational, autonomous self-assertion.

The Importance of the Family as Story

By owning, aiming, and sharing their power, families perform the maternal and moral work children require if they are to grow happily and contribute responsibly to their communities. But families are more than nurseries; they perform crucial work for the adults within them as well. Because family relationships endure over time, they provide a means for *maintaining* the identities that earlier configurations of the family once forged. Family members, like old friends, are in a position to know us well and to treat us in accordance with that knowledge; we in turn respond to that treatment in ways that reinforce their perception. In this way children have an ongoing impact on the selves of their parents—an impact different in degree but as great in intensity as that of a spouse or same-sex partner. Maintaining the self is an essential function that our intimates help us to perform, but their participation is dangerous, particularly when their perception of us is negative. If, for example, our family wrongly regards us as stupid or untrustworthy, we are apt not only to become so, but to remain so.

But we need not. We can instead affirm certain aspects of our relationships with our families and repudiate others—as we affirm or repudiate other centrally important, identity-constitutive features of our lives—in an ongoing process of what the philosopher Margaret Urban Walker has called strong moral self-definition.[21] That is, we can use decisions we must make about our lives—about our medical care, for example—to set a new course for ourselves or to confirm the goodness of an existing course. In this way, families contribute to the continued moral growth of their adult members. While opportunities for strong moral self-definition are not restricted to families, small-scale, emotionally dense contexts are ready occasions for such a process. We'll have more to say about strong moral self-definition later.

The involvement of family in maintaining one's self-identity, however, goes beyond actual interchanges with one's family members. Of equal importance is one's place in the family's story. Families link us to a particular past and particular future, as they root us in their traditions and affirm for us what is worth living and working for. The family reconfigures as the people within it grow, but the story that is lived out within the successive configurations preserves its continuity. This ongoing tale, to which each individual's life-story contributes a narrative thread, makes an enormous contribution both to our sense of who we are, and to our sense of why it matters who we are.

There would seem to be no better way of illustrating this point than by actually telling stories. Imagine a woman suddenly stricken by selective amnesia. She can remember everything except her family. She no longer remembers her husband, or her former husband, or her current struggles to help her stepchildren adjust to her; she has no recollection of her sister in California or her brother in Africa; she has forgotten most of her childhood because she cannot remember the traditions, customs, values, or tenor of life of her family of origin. She steps on a rag rug in her bedroom without recalling that she watched her aunt braid it when she was a child; it is now just a rug. She does not understand her trick of smiling brightly when she is unhappy, having no memory of her mother's similar response to sorrow. Her belief in God no longer contains the doubts once introduced by her husband's agnosticism. Who is she, now that she has come unmoored from her familial past and from the present?

Or think of a Southern family of decayed aristocrats—a family now in tatters but still proud of its antebellum past. The women drink too much and the men, after four years at Harvard, brood silently in dusty, small-town law offices. To this family a son is born. Were he to grow up among his people, his personality, his character, and his personal story would add their texture to the Faulknerian novel that is the fabric not only of his day-to-day life, but of his very self. But fate decrees otherwise. Through whatever mechanism you care to imagine, the boy is taken at birth to a prosperous midwestern farming community, where he is reared by a family whose life revolves around church activities and the farm machinery dealership that is the family business. The fabric of his life is now a novel written by Garrison Keillor, and while he may well grow up to rebel against his provincial and corn-fed existence, he does it as a part of *this* novel, not the other.

The moral of these stories? Put rather bluntly, in the manner of good morals, it is this: families make us who we are. Through their narrative structures we live out our own particular stories, and as they share their power with us we come to self-knowledge and self-respect. They are, then, of *instrumental* value to us. The family's maternal work is also instrumentally valuable—it is a means of achieving the goods of protection, nurturing, and socialization. But what is there about the family that we value for its own sake?

The Family as an End in Itself

John Rawls has a concept that comes in handy here—the notion of a primary good. A primary good is a thing "that every rational man is presumed to want," such as health, intelligence, security, a means of support. Goods of this kind "normally have a use whatever a person's rational plan of life" and for that reason are means to some other end. But for Rawls, the most important primary good—self-respect—is an end in itself. He says self-respect is "not so much a part of any rational plan of life as the sense that one's plan is worth carrying out."[22] We have already implied that familial love, as the flooring upon which we take our first steps toward independence, promotes self-respect. But the fact is that the family has a value beyond its ability to promote self-respect, or to give people a personal identity, or physical care, or social and moral education, or any of a number of other things worth having. This fact is easier to understand if we think of what it would be like if someone "loved" us only to help us attain one of these other goods—let's say, as Rawls is keen on it, the good of self-respect.

Imagine a struggling young singer whose debut with a major opera company is a disaster: despite his best efforts, his opening night performance is so bad that the director fires him. Yet singing is his life. He has no confidence in himself, and if it weren't for his bride of six months, who has unbounded faith in him, he would have no reason to go on. But he does go on, and after years of further struggle, during which he endures rejection after rejection and his self-esteem is at its nadir, he auditions again—this time for the Metropolitan Opera Company—and lands the role of Tamino in *The Magic Flute.* With fear and trepidation and with his wife to cheer him on, he throws himself body and soul into rehearsal, and his opening night is brilliant. The audience roars its adulation, the rest of the cast applauds him, and the next day the critics are raving over their new discovery. That day his wife takes him out to lunch and breaks the news that she is leaving him. She has been having an affair with another man, but as an act of love felt she should help the singer to get back his confidence before she brought up the question of a divorce.

The singer sadly replies, "But if you loved me only to give me confidence, then you didn't really love me at all."

We seek love for its own sake, and not just for what it can do for us. The singer was right to suggest that if love is used only instrumentally, it is ersatz love. It's one thing for a relationship to enhance self-respect, or to provide a career boost, or to gain entrée into a particular social set if these benefits are "by the way," but it is quite another if the relationship becomes solely a means to such ends. The betrayal of the singer—quite apart from the question of infidelity—consisted in his wife's viewing their marriage wholly in terms of its usefulness to him.

What if, conversely, he had sought to love his wife as a means of helping himself along? What if his motto had been, "I'll feel much better about myself if I love another"? If feeling better about himself had been his primary goal, then he would have been acting not out of love for his wife, but out of love for himself. This kind of instrumental use of love is incoherent. Love's fundamental presupposition is that the beloved is to be cherished, not used.

The Family's Role in Times of Illness

Families, then, are valuable for all kinds of reasons: they protect, socialize, and care for us; they forge and help maintain our identities; they give us our first lessons in morality; they are good in and of themselves. But what is their special usefulness in times of illness? This book, after all, is an exploration of two systems of dealing with illness—that of the family, and that of medicine. What happens when these two systems interact?

For one thing, even when the illness is so severe as to require professional assistance, families are actively involved in the ill person's care. For another, families make decisions about that care if the person is too young or too ill to decide such matters for herself. Both functions are commonly accepted, and we will have more to say about them later. Here, however, we want to explore a third and less well understood service families provide for the seriously ill: that of domesticating the illness—overcoming the alienation we experience when we can no longer take for granted the smooth functioning of our bodies.

Injuries and illnesses—even comparatively minor ones—have the effect of estranging us from ourselves. They create a *Verfremdungseffekt*, to use a term of Bertolt Brecht's—an "alienation effect" that distances us from the ordinary and the familiar features of life, making us profoundly uncomfortable. We are in foreign territory when our body ceases to function properly; not only our bodies, but also the projects, surroundings, and routines that make up the course of our day are temporarily or permanently estranged from us. And because these projects, surroundings, and routines have their own part to play in our identity, in their absence we experience a more precarious hold on ourselves than we do in ordinary times.[23] Even in cases of mild illness, the old-fashioned inquiry after one's health—"Are you quite yourself again?"—bears witness to the connection between identity and well-being.

Where the illness or injury is severe, the alienation effect is correspondingly greater, and so is the threat this effect poses to the usual self. That self, expressed in the myriad little intentions and purposes of daily life, is now

45

in danger of disintegrating, yet is amazingly difficult to give up. The physician-philosopher Eric Cassell tells of a young woman who was flung from a motorcycle with terrible force, slamming into a concrete barrier and then onto the highway. Her first deliberate act was to pull her skirt down over her badly broken legs. She was not able to let go of her usual "myself" and attempted, with that gesture, to protect it.[24] But she could only domesticate the catastrophe to a limited degree; beyond that, she would need her family to help her.

In the midst of all the strangeness of illness or injury, alienated from ourselves and from the ongoing ordinariness of things, we can turn to our families for orientation to our new reality. The family's mechanisms for maintaining selves are never so useful as here, when we first begin to guage the effect of bodily catastrophe on who we are. Our domestic intimates can help us reclaim our selves by providing a fixed and familiar point of reference for us as we struggle with the disaster. When the illness is chronic, family members do the same thing over time, quelling the effect of self-alienation by the very ordinariness of their own personalities.

The Family in the Hospital

If an illness is serious enough to require hospitalization or a nursing home, the person suffering it not only experiences an erosion of self, but also the alienation that comes from being uprooted from domestic surroundings and thrust into a foreign environment with foreign routines and a foreign code of conscience. When one's hold on one's identity is already attenuated by physical trauma, it is disturbing and frightening to find oneself in a total institution that is not only un-familiar but also structurally resistant to being familiar-ized. By their very nature, institutions that care for the sick—particularly acute-care institutions—are not designed to offer the comforts of home. Indeed, they subsume not only individual patients but also their families into a foreign terrain. Or, to put it another way, they domesticate families unto themselves.

NOT FAMILY-FRIENDLY

Mario Pisani suspects he is having a heart attack and is brought to the emergency room of a first-rate hospital providing excellent care. Alienation from his family begins immediately. Mario is taken for examination to a cubicle too small to accommodate his wife and three teenaged children. Then Maddalena Pisani and the children go to the admissions office, which typically has only two chairs, to take care of the paperwork. Meanwhile, Mario is being admitted to the hospital.

The hospital's visiting hours are from two in the afternoon until eight at night. Those hours are chosen because they don't conflict with the day's most intense hospital activity, which occurs in the morning. But because Dr. Jackson makes her rounds then, when the family isn't present, Maddalena Pisani has no first-hand information about the attending physician's visit. By the time she sees her husband that evening, he's forgotten some of the details, and in any case doesn't feel well enough to give her a blow-by-blow description.

Dr. Jackson, for her part, considers the process by which she elicits Mr. Pisani's informed consent to treatment to be private; she has an obligation to ensure the visit is confidential so that if Mr. Pisani chooses, he can tell her things he doesn't want his wife or children to know. But this means any decisions regarding treatment must be made in a fragmented way. Dr. Jackson understands how frustrating this is for Mrs. Pisani and tries conscientiously to keep the rest of the Pisanis informed about major developments, but the best way to achieve this is to set up a group meeting, and her busy schedule permits fewer of these than she'd like.

She makes a special effort a few days later to come back when Mrs. Pisani and the children are there, so she can explain to them all why Mr. Pisani needs a bypass operation. She's very good at this—she neither confuses them with technical language nor frightens them unduly by an exhaustive recital of all the things that can go wrong, but at the same time she's careful to give them a realistic understanding of what it will be like. The operation proceeds without incident. When it is over, Mrs. Pisani enters the critical care unit to see her husband connected to a machine, with tubes coming out of his nose and throat, and other tubes dripping fluids into both his arms. His color is bad and he is in a stupor. She has never seen him like this, corpselike and made of marble instead of flesh. One flesh. Husband and wife, she thinks, are one flesh, and she remembers the comfortable contours of his body beside her at night these many years. This body lying before her now, though, has nothing to do with her flesh—nothing to do with *her*. She is glad that he is asleep so she does not have to touch him, and when she realizes that she is glad it distresses her very much.

Mr. Pisani makes good progress and is soon transferred to the general cardiac floor. As the hospital stay lengthens, he learns a new system of etti-quette—one that confuses his family and tends to estrange him from them. Mr. Pisani is ordinarily a pleasant but positive person, happy to negotiate differences with others and used to asserting himself when he must. But he finds that in a hospital, the strategies of negotiation and assertion don't work as well as cooperation and manipulation do. He finds that if he gets along with the staff by being passive and grateful he'll get better care than if he complains or confronts; there is something about the prone position that invites care. He is shrewd enough to understand this, so when one evening his dinner arrives cold and an hour late, he hushes his wife as she begins to protest. She is taken aback by this and feels lonely again; she and her husband don't even share the same life-strategies any more. At least, they don't right now. She wonders what the future will be like.

As if all that weren't bad enough, Mr. Pisani begins to adapt to hospital life by bonding with a new group—his roommates and their visitors. He takes more of an interest in the goings-on in his room than he does in his daughter's day at school or his co-workers' news from the factory; the life he sees from his hospital bed is more present to him than the world outside. In these and countless other ways he becomes subtly estranged from the values and relationships that in health seemed quite important.[25]

The un-familiarity of the hospital, then, is at least as hard on his family as it is on Mario Pisani. Unfortunately, at the very moment when his heart disease and the hospital environment join forces to estrange him from his family, he needs his wife and children most especially, for the bonds of love and shared history between them that are now being eroded are the very bonds that will help him get well. Study after study has demonstrated that patients who have intimates they can turn to for affection, affirmation, empathy, and assistance are more likely to survive heart attacks and major surgery than patients who do not. According to a study of 1,368 heart patients published recently in the *Journal of the American Medical Association*, those who had no spouse or intimate friend were three times as likely to die within five years of diagnosis as those who had. A study in

Alameda County, California, tracking thousands of patients over a nine-year period, came to the same conclusion. And research conducted at the University of Nebraska School of Medicine involving 256 healthy, elderly people found that those in intimate relationships had lower cholesterol and uric acid levels in their blood and better immune function.[26]

These studies shouldn't surprise us; there is a strong connection between our emotional and our physical well-being. Such findings also testify to the robustness of family ties; bonds between family members usually endure to nurture even those who have undergone prolonged encounters with the health care system. This suggests that medicine has a powerful reason for taking families seriously, and not just as aids to making patients more "comfortable." The very health outcomes that medicine is set up to promote—the values internal to its own practice, so to speak—often cry out for health-care professionals to make active use of family ties. Instead, the health care system estranges patients like Mr. Pisani from the relationships that are most fundamental to emotional well-being, thereby creating a potential for even greater damage than that already inflicted by lack of oxygen to the heart muscle.

Why Families Are Hard to See

Because of its effect on the patient's health, this estrangement from the family should be of concern to health-care givers. It makes good medical sense for those involved in a patient's care to do what they can to strengthen rather than erode the ties that bind patients and their intimates. Nurses, who get to know both patient and family well, tend to be sensitive to this need; the hospital's social workers, who are trained to think in terms of group dynamics, are as a rule also sympathetic to it. But the physicians and hospital administrators who structure the delivery of care have not been educated to see the significance for healing of the bond between patient and family. This is not to say they don't pay lip service to it. They do. But because they aren't thinking of what families are really like (even though they themselves usually live in them), there is something formulaic and uninformed about their routine invocations of the patient's family. And so, instead of harnessing the family's healthgiving potential—its power to domesticate illness and restore to the patient his sense of self—hospitals tend to subject the family to the sorts of stresses and strains the Pisanis encountered.

That hospitals do not foster the conditions under which patients' ties to their families are nourished and strengthened isn't to be wondered at. Institutional realities are such that doctors sometimes have a hard time relating in a human way with the patients themselves, let alone with their families. When medicine became very good at curing disease and saving lives, it also became very technological. At that point, physicians were offered a strong temptation to abstract the indicators of disease from the living patient—to regard the readouts on machines as the clearest expression of the patient's state of health. They succumbed to the temptation, and were not the only ones to do so. In neonatal intensive care units, for example, where very premature babies struggle for life, their parents soon learn to attach great significance to these figures, even though they have only the haziest notion of what all the indicators, taken together, reveal about their babies' conditions. "How can we blame them for focusing on the numbers?" asks one of the doctors. "That's what we talk to them about; that's what we've taught them."[27] That's what they've learned themselves.

To counteract this tendency to focus on the numbers, many medical schools are beginning to institute programs in the medical humanities. Along with physiology and anatomy textbooks, med students now also read Tolstoy's "The Death of Ivan Ilych" and William Carlos Williams's "The Use of Force," as a way of helping them understand just what kind of animal they will be taking care of when they graduate. Healing, they are told, is more complex than vending: the doctor cannot simply produce a solution to a specific malfunction, in exchange for money. That is, it's not an illness that must be treated, but an embodied, desiring, thinking, and feeling person. Doctors will make serious mistakes if they don't understand that illness occurs in a human being with a history and a set of life-circumstances.

An example. In her novel *Other Women's Children,* Perri Klass tells of a third-year medical student's first night on duty in the emergency room of a teaching hospital in Boston. Jasper is conscientious, eager to please, hard-working—in fact, he is so conscientious that he takes an hour to examine his second patient. His attending physician, whose job is to supervise him, sees the nurse's note that the patient is a two-year-old with an upper respiratory infection and wonders why Jasper needs an hour to diagnose a cold. When Jasper emerges from the examining cubicle where the mother and child are waiting, he presents his diagnosis to "the attending" in unbelievable detail:

> the age, the weight, the height, every detail of every sniffle. "Four days prior to this emergency-room visit, the mother first noted some slightly increased congestion, worsening in the evening. There was no associated rhinorrhea or cough, and no other symptoms at that time, including no fever, no vomiting, no diarrhea. The cough developed three days prior to this visit, and is described as dry, not productive of sputum." And on and on. And all I could think [writes the attending] was here is this young man of normal intelligence, and his brain has been so bent out of shape that he is not capable of saying, "The kid has a cold."[28]

But when the attending accompanies Jasper back into the cubicle to check his diagnosis, she sees immediately what Jasper, for all his exhaustive thoroughness, has overlooked. In hospital slang, the little two-year-old girl is "toaster-headed"—her head is almost square, flattened especially in the back. She is the size of a scrawny one-year-old, her chest is marked with four surgical scars, and she is wheezing. These are all indications that the child was extremely premature, which in turn means that she probably spent a long time on a ventilator, and *that* means lungs "like an eighty-year-old chain smoker's." The scars indicate heart surgery. The child may or may not have a cold, but she surely has bronchopulmonary dysplasia, a lung disease that is seen in children who have spent a lot of time in infancy on the ventilator.

Well, Jasper is young, and his attending will teach him to see more than the symptoms of the cold that are the reason for the visit to the emergency room in the first place. Medical students are now being taught to see the *whole* person, history and all. But we want to take this move one step further, to ask doctors to learn to see the whole person *in relationship with others*. If, that is, a cold must be situated—set into the historical context of the person who suffers from it—so too must the person be situated within the nest of relationships where she lives her life.

Taking Families Seriously

To some extent, of course, doctors already do this. Pediatricians, for example, can't help but notice the dependence that is such a strong feature of the bond between a baby and its parents. But when an illness is cast in terms of its meaning for the family, it is usually the instrumental nature of the relationship that is recognized: the baby's relationship to its parents is useful because they can provide consent for treatment on the baby's behalf; the patient's relationship with an identical twin is useful because the twin has the kidney that can be transplanted with the least risk of rejection into the patient; the existence of a spouse is useful for a cardiovascular patient because nonmarried patients are at increased risk of death in the setting of coronary heart disease. The family, like a surgical procedure or a prescription drug, is one among many medical resources the physician draws upon to heal the patient.

But to say this not really to appreciate the fact that patients come attached to families—it is only to make use of that fact. Just as doctors learn to see the patient as a person in his own right and not merely a collection of vital signs, or merely an opportunity for healing, so too, we argue, they can learn to see families as valuable in themselves, and not merely as items in the doctor's dispensary. It is sometimes said that over the last twenty years the great contribution of bioethics to medical practice has been to remind doctors that they may not use patients for their own ends, no matter how benevolent those ends might be, but must rather respect patients as persons in their own right, who must be allowed to determine for themselves what shape their lives will take. Similarly, doctors can learn that families should not be used solely for the ends of healing, but must be honored in their own right. They can learn to be mindful of the fact that families, like persons, have their own value and integrity—that they are places where people are cherished. The fact that family members can make decisions for us when we are very ill is really beside the point; we want them there not for what they can do for us but because they love us.

THE HOSPITAL VISITOR'S POLICY

Jean M. is gray-haired and quietly dressed, a secretary who has been with her publishing firm so long that people say of her, "Jean *is* Coronet Publishing." She was divorced fifteen years ago, when her children were in college; both her son and her daughter live on the West Coast now. We are lunching with her in a little Manhattan restaurant where the manicotti is excellent and the tables are gay with blue and white checked cloths. As the waiter brings the espresso, Jean says, "It wasn't all that long after the divorce. I hadn't been feeling particularly well all week, and then I got an earache.

My boss was worried about me, and kept telling me to go to the doctor, but I wouldn't. I remember that Saturday afternoon he came over to my house, and took one look at me, and drove me to the hospital himself. He saved my life, you know. I had meningitis. I almost died from it—I would have, if he hadn't interfered.

"They took good care of me at the hospital, I guess. But what I couldn't stand was their visitor's policy. I was in the Intensive Care Unit for almost a week, and in those days they were very strict about ICU visits. No more than fifteen minutes at a time, and definitely family only. Well, it was my lover I needed then, but they wouldn't let him in, no matter how hard he tried to talk them around. He was there every day, but I didn't know it. You know who they let in? My ex-husband. What made them think I'd want to see my ex-husband?"

We shook our heads and sipped our espresso meditatively. The lunch crowd had thinned considerably, and the restaurant had taken on its afternoon look.

"I'll tell you what it was." Jean reached across the white and blue cloth for the check. "It's not just that they didn't understand who my family was. The real trouble was that they forgot why families *matter*."[29]

Chapter Three

An Ethics for Families

A FEW YEARS AGO THE PHILOSOPHER JOHN HARDWIG was explaining Kant's moral theories to a classroom of undergraduate students. He had gotten to the passage where Kant argues that only actions done from duty are morally worthy—if you're merely following your own natural inclinations you haven't done anything that matters from a moral point of view. At this point a young woman demanded, "Is Kant saying that if I sleep with my boyfriend, I should sleep with him out of a sense of duty?" Hardwig's response: "And when you're through, you should tell him that you would have done the same for anyone in his situation."[1] It seems that some theories of even the greatest moral philosophers don't work very well when we try to apply them to our intimate relationships. What's morally important about our interactions with those whom we love isn't easily captured by impersonal accounts of our duties to others.

This is worth thinking about. Most of us have a pretty good sense of what's required of us in our interactions with colleagues, clients, fellow citizens, and others whom we don't know well: we understand about fairness, honesty, minding our own business, living up to our bargains, and so on.

And we also know why, in the abstract, we owe these people respectful treatment—we (or most of us, anyway) have general notions about the dignity and inherent worth of all human beings.

Similarly, we have a pretty good sense of what's required of doctors in their interactions with patients: we understand that physicians are supposed to respect patients' autonomy, that their first responsibility is to help the patient get better, if that's possible, or to ease the patient's suffering if nothing more can be done. And we also know why, in the abstract, we value what physicians do for their patients: medicine holds out the promise of keeping us healthy, of making us well when we have been sick, and of keeping us alive when, without its ministrations, we'd be quite dead. And it has other promises as well: to give us children when we can't produce them on our own, to give us back our youth when our breasts have started to sag and our heads become hairless, to soothe us when life challenges our ability to cope on our own.

In short, we understand a fair amount about ordinary morality and about the more localized version of morality that is medical ethics. What we don't understand very well, though, is how morality works within the context of families. As Professor Hardwig's student suggests, it seems funny to invoke justice under the sheets, strange to stand on your rights with someone you care about.

Our task in this chapter is to identify some of the features of family life that distinguish it from other spheres, and show how these features are morally significant. In doing so, we hope to better understand and ease the tensions between families and the medical profession. While the full dimensions of the troubled relationship between the two systems can't be understood without the perspectives of other disciplines—psychology, sociology, history, economics, and law have obvious contributions to make—the fundamental problem is a moral one: a clash between two different systems of value. This being the case, the solution must be fundamentally a moral one as well, so to find the solution we work with a set of moral ideas.

If the bioethics revolution is pictured as a conversation between general theories of morality worked out by philosophers and the ethical traditions of medicine, then what is happening in this book is that a third party is now joining that conversation—a theory of the special moral values of intimacy, in particular, of familial relationships. As we will see, the moral notions guiding intimacy are importantly different from those informing either general or medical ethics; the relationships among the three have not been often or well described.

Leading Ideas in General Theories of Morality

Contemporary ethical views are built on a variety of fundamental ideas, not all of which fit together in any tidy sort of way: God's will, or, less directly, God's ordering of the natural world; basic and inalienable rights; the consequences of what we do. Although these theories are different and can lead to widely divergent moral conclusions, they do share some common themes.

One such theme might be called *individualism.* Our sense of what's right and wrong tends very much to be a matter of the impact of what we do on other, individual people. The broad ethical theories—particularly those that most heavily influence our contemporary life—aren't directly concerned with groups or collectivities of any kind.

This hasn't been useless, by any means. To take just one example, individualism provides a perspective from which to see clearly the evils of discrimination as they are revealed in slavery, sexism, or racism. Class, gender, or race, this perspective argues, are not facts about individuals that carry any moral weight.

In dismissing the significance of groups of which one is a part, however, we can miss important dimensions of moral experience. Consider Jane King, a young African American woman trying hard to climb the corporate ladder. If she's earned a promotion but doesn't receive it because she is a woman, or because she is black, the moral verdict is clear: her rights have been violated, and she's entitled to redress. Yet the individualistic focus that is so prominent in our ethical (and legal) tradition has made it difficult to give a good account of why not only she, but also the group she belongs to, is entitled to redress. The notion of a group, as opposed to an individual, being a subject of harm is hard to make sense of from an individualistic perspective. The idea that Jane King deserves special attention in the job market because of the moral history of her race and gender is much more controversial than the idea that she shouldn't be discriminated against because of her race or gender. The claim that, for example, her ability to bear and nurse a child entitles her to special treatment in the workplace—say, special accommodations concerning leaves and promotions—is so controversial that even people who regard themselves as feminists disagree about it. Jane King's situation and our social response to it are influenced by our history of moral individualism, and give rise to what Martha Minow calls "dilemmas of difference."[2] How can we take proper account of the differences among us without reinforcing patterns of unfair discrimination that may be based on just those differences?

The major players within contemporary moral theory also share a commitment to *impartiality*. "Each to count as one and none for more than one," as the classical utilitarian thinker Jeremy Bentham pithily put it. His point was that everyone's interests have the same claim on our attention when we're deciding public policy or individual practice. This is impartial because no one is favored. Again, this insight makes a great deal of sense when we are focused on the life of our public institutions and our interactions with strangers. It's part of the reason why a rational person would accept being governed by moral considerations: her interests count as much as anyone else's, and while she gets no special privileges, that's fair enough, because no one else does either.

Even the most ardent promoter of a particular cause or group of people might admit (at least if pressed hard enough) that there are limits to the amount of special pleading that's morally permissible on the group's behalf; an impartial moral system might well show us just where those limits lie. For example, a theory like Bentham's, in which morality consists of acting in ways that tend to promote the happiness of everyone impartially considered, might well allow a certain place for friendship, love, and loyalty; within bounds, the presence of such things improves our lives, makes all of us happier than we'd otherwise be.[3] But pressed too far, personal loyalties start to backfire and produce more unhappiness on the whole than happiness—they produce, for example, an unwillingness to raise taxes for public schools because your own children attend private academies, or a readiness to hand out favors to friends and relatives once you are sworn in as mayor. At that point, loyalties must give way to a more direct concern for the common good, on the "each to count as one" principle. While it's not at all easy to show that special loyalties can be accommodated within an impartialist framework—at least, not if the loyalty is genuine—impartialist theories certainly make an effort to show how all of our moral behavior, the "private" as well as the "public," can be captured within a single, unified system.[4]

The third important feature about ordinary moral theory (as Hardwig explained to the young woman with the boyfriend) is that it is strongly *universalizable*. That is, its most fundamental directives for action—for example, "Thou shalt not kill"—are not directed to particular persons, nor are they directed to particular situations. They are intended to guide the behavior of anyone, regardless of who they are, in all relevant circumstances. While the class of actors and the class of actions can be specified sharply—as in "for a limited period of time, licensed psychiatrists may detain people they suspect of being dangerous" they cannot single out individuals. "Jill may detain Jack on Thursday, June 4," is not a moral principle—although it might of course *follow* from a moral principle, if Jill were a psychiatrist, and Jack dangerous.

There's a sense in which universalizability is such an obvious feature of anything that could count as a moral judgment that it isn't worth discussing. Logically, this is simply to say that if we were to judge a certain action or policy as wrong, and another action or policy arose that was identical to the first in all morally relevant respects, we would have to judge it wrong also—or, if we think that the second policy is acceptable, we would have to change our assessment of the first.

But much hinges on what we count as morally relevant. If you move to a high enough level of abstraction, you can find relevant similarities among all kinds of actions. For example, there must be thousands of situations that could be described abstractly by the statement, "X is telling a lie." But because many of the morally important features of a situation take their meaning from highly specific elements that overlap in very particular configurations, the exact situation of the lie isn't very likely to crop up again—in fact, it may be quite unique. To whom was the lie told? For what reason? What other values would have been violated in this particular context had the truth been told? Was there a history to the interaction between X and the recipient of the lie that has a legitimate bearing on the case? And so on.

Margaret Walker has explored this question of the abstract and the particular by discussing a family's decision to put Grandmother into a nursing home.[5] While this is clearly a moral decision, she points out that some of the very features that give that particular family's relationships their own special character—for example, how the wife and husband in question understand their marriage, where it has come from, where it is going, and what it means to their lives—also bear importantly on the decision. That these features are so individual—even individuating, helping to make *this very relationship* what it is—doesn't mean that they apply only to the particular decision about Grandmother. If a similar question were to arise about Grandfather, it's hard to imagine that similar considerations wouldn't be at least relevant to the family's deliberations.

The stress on universalizability, impartiality, and individualism encourages an ethical perspective that tends to shun anything that seems too idiosyncratic, too contingent, too parochial. It aspires to what has been styled a "view from nowhere."[6] This perspective helps us understand why judgments and actions that are mired in particularity are likely to go wrong. They are too arbitrary and inadequately sensitive to the need to justify rationally and defend publicly what one does. However, the "view from nowhere" has also distorted the significance of many of the features of human life—the inevitable importance of the specific details of each of our experiences, our connectedness with special others, and the distinctive needs and vulnerabilities that arise from these parts of our lives. This is no small matter, as the personal and private aspects of our lives are crucial to who we are and why we care to be in the world at all.[7]

Medical Ethics

The traditional ethics of medicine shares with the more general tradition of ethics a primary concern with individuals; in fact, medicine's traditions are almost obsessively individualistic. Even in the current climate of massive cost and heavily restricted access to medical services—trends that raise real concerns about justice—many physicians think it's flatly wrong to take broader communal concerns into account when making treatment decisions for their patients. Some even think it's their duty to resist the socially imposed structures (health maintenance organizations, for example) that attempt to control health care costs by reviewing and restricting the therapies to which patients have access.[8]

But of course medicine is not ethically devoted to *all* individuals: the traditional idea is that it's only those people who have succeeded in convincing a physician to begin a "doctor-patient" relationship who are the subject of special moral concern. Thus, the traditional medical ethics is not at all impartial—quite the contrary. Nor is it triggered simply by a realization of the vulnerability and need of ill people; rather, it is a contractual ethics in which all special duties flow from a relationship freely entered into by willing participants. Because medicine is individualistic, and selectively individualistic at that, it tends to favor those who are powerful enough to enter into the doctor-patient relationship. It favors those with more rather than less money, education, social standing. And because it focuses on persons rather than groups, it isn't easily responsive to systemic patterns of injustice within its practice. Instead, it tends to repeat these patterns—as, for example, when women are systematically excluded from participation in clinical trials of an experimental drug or technology, or when the disproportionate amount of child or elder care demanded of women forces them into part-time jobs with no health insurance benefits.[9]

Medical ethics is also narrow in focus compared to common, everyday morality: a physician's duties are specific, rather than general, being confined to such things as curing illness or injury, easing suffering, and preventing disease. In addition, the physician is traditionally obligated to refrain from using his or her power over the vulnerable patient in ways that would be harmful or exploitative: confidentiality is to be observed, sexual relationships (and, by implication, other forms of intimacy) are ruled out.

Medical ethics, again unlike general ethics, is grounded in a social practice—in the particular, culture-specific traditions of the profession, running all the way back to the Hippocratic Oath. Appeals to tradition don't serve as a very strong basis for ethical conduct, however. "We've always done it that way" doesn't tell physicians whether they *ought* always to have done it that way, still less whether they ought to continue doing it that way now. Contemporary medical ethics—or bioethics—is something of a marriage between its own traditional values and values more widely agreed upon in everyday life, such as beneficence, respect for autonomy, justice, and fidelity.[10]

In a pluralistic culture, these principles are particularly attractive as guides to practical action because they can be derived from many of the more general moral traditions. It doesn't matter if your morality is founded on the teachings of Jesus or the maxim that you should do the greatest good for the greatest number, since either moral source will support the importance of justice, beneficence, and fidelity. Since they at least appear to be compatible with traditional medical values, these principles are also available to guide physicians' practice. Broadly, they secure an ethical focus on the interests of the patient; at finer levels, they continue to support such long-standing ideals as confidentiality and fidelity to the patient.

At the same time, these principles guide doctors in correcting traditional practices that now strike most of us as wrong. Perhaps the outstanding such practice is *paternalism*, the notion that physicians ought to decide what is best for the patient, rather than letting the patient determine this for herself. A newfound respect for the autonomy of patients has put paternalism, formerly a pervasive part of American medicine, at least somewhat on the defensive, without undermining the ethical bedrock that physicians are to serve the patient's good.

This is not to claim that, once medical ethics opened itself up to correction with the help of more general moral principles, everything was strengthened and nothing disturbed. Consider the upheaval that the principle of social justice is now creating among physicians. Doctor Gillespie, who has been in family practice for nearly a third of a century, has very little use for health maintenance organizations or other forms of managed care intended to control medical costs. "I know we've got a health care crisis on our hands in this country," he growls, entering an order for kidney dialysis into the chart of an eighty-nine-year-old patient. "I know we're spending too much money on these services and not enough on education or housing or crime in the streets, and if Congress passes reform legislation so everybody has access to care, we'll be spending even more. But I can't be worrying about that—it's not my job to look down the road and see where we'll end up if the spending isn't slowed down somehow. Somebody else is going to have to tackle that problem. My job is to do the very best I can for each one of my patients, and the cost be damned."

It may be helpful to think of the recent history of medical ethics as maintaining a steady course of increasing ethical complexity. The traditional physician had, at base, one moral rule to observe: benefit the patient. Contemporary physicians have for several years now been wrestling with the additional claim that they must take their patients seriously. They are to see patients as active decisionmakers who can often determine their medical interests for themselves, and who won't always opt for courses of action the physician approves. Matters became even messier when questions of justice in the allocation of medical resources become too pressing for physicians to sidestep: they are being asked to take *society* seriously. Considerations of social justice now make a compelling argument that doctors must try to balance the interests of patients with the interests of the country at large.

To this melange of moral requirements that medicine faces we must now add yet one more: taking *families* seriously. Doing this will involve a number of challenges. How will not only physicians, but all interested parties, recognize which families are competent to be involved in decisionmaking? How should all those involved in the care of the sick balance family interests versus individual interests? How do we all resolve conflicts between provider integrity and familial integrity? Considerations stemming from the moral significance of intimacy, as well as of justice, demand that everyone do their best here as well.

The Ethics of the Intimate

Doing our best here isn't a matter of simply adding families and stirring. The complexities introduced by paying moral attention to families are of a different order from those that were introduced when, with the infusion of contemporary moral theory, traditional medical ethics became what is now often called bioethics. That infusion merely required a stronger commitment to the *impersonal* point of view that had been governing medical ethics all along. Sensitivity to familial complexities, on the other hand, requires a willingness to make conceptual and practical room for the *personal* point of view as well.[11] If individualism, impartiality, and universalizability are the leading features of general theories of morality, the morality of intimacy can be characterized rather differently. Its leading features are collectivity, favoritism, particularity, nonconsensuality, and a premodern sensibility.

Collectivity

Oddly enough, although family values are personal, the morality of families tends to be less individualistic than those of either the general run of ethics or its bioethical variations. Actions and rules are often assessed in terms of their impact on the family overall, in a manner that's hard to reduce to the interests of individual family members. This point may be clearest if family traditions are considered. Some practice or theme in a family's life—returning to the same cottage every summer, or honoring Polish ancestry—may have value to a particular family member not simply because summer at the cottage or observing Polish customs makes that person's life richer, but because he knows that the rest of the family feels the same way.

This interactive valuing, whereby a tradition or practice takes on a distinctive significance for each because it has a distinctive significance for all, involves some degree of collective responsibility. Painting the cottage or making an effort to speak Polish with one's grandmother might be something of a chore, but in keeping up these traditions one participates in the continuing process of group self-definition.

Consider a sports-minded family with a very talented ten-year-old gymnast. They might well devote collective effort and energy toward helping the child excel, even though this means that not every member of the family gets what might otherwise be considered a fair share of the available resources. While such situations surely are dangerous—one can easily imagine how they might degenerate into a kind of abuse of other family members—the danger does not itself entail immorality; a family's giving a preferential share of what it has to a particular member, because of her particular vulnerabilities or talents, is not necessarily wrong, and may indeed be not only permitted, but obligatory.

Favoritism

This brings us directly to another distinguishing feature of familial ethics: whereas medical ethics strongly favors patients, and ethics in general bids us not to play favorites at all, family ethics favors other family members—and does so in a strong and distinct way.

Contrast the basic rationale for favoring patients with the situation in families. Physicians favor patients because patients are often vulnerable due to disease or injury. Even if they are not, they still must make themselves vulnerable to the physician, physically and often emotionally, if the physician's expertise is to be of any use. Patients must trust physicians with a precious thing—their own bodies—and, while their informed and critical involvement in their care is important, sooner or later patients must simply believe that the physician knows what she's doing. In order to secure patients' trust and defend their vulnerability, their interests are placed first.

But note how instrumental this mutual loyalty is. We don't so much value it in itself, as for what it may help us get—a safe and useful medical encounter. Familial favoritism, by contrast, is not merely instrumental. While we surely make ourselves vulnerable to others in the family, these others don't favor us solely to keep themselves from exploiting our vulnerability. Both letting ourselves be vulnerable to those we love and being prized by our loved ones over others are part of what it *means* to us to be loved. Such things are valuable, not just for what they buy us, but for what they are.

From a common sense perspective, the value of being loved for yourself has great and obvious force. But this isn't an insight that has been thoroughly integrated into current discussions of medical ethics, and for that reason it's worth pursuing.

MISS PYM PLAYS FAVORITES

Miss Amelia Pym is a forty-five-year-old schoolteacher who has lived in the sleepy little town of Bishop, Ohio, all her life. Since the death of her parents many years ago she has kept house for her brother Harry, who drifted from one job to the next until his addiction to alcohol became so overpowering that he succumbed completely. Always resistant to treatment, he has divided his time for the last five years between the tavern in the next block and his living room at home. There he sits watching television in the evenings with his martini shaker close by, until he falls asleep in his chair. A year ago Harry was diagnosed as having a particularly vicious form of leukemia. He was taken to Columbus, where a bone marrow transplant was attempted. Because it failed, Harry has at the most only six months to live. Blood transfusions will keep him going for a while, but finally they too will fail.

Miss Amelia Pym has O-negative blood, which means that she is a universal donor. She has been giving Harry pints of her blood as frequently as his physician allows it, for she is very fond of Harry in spite of everything, and will miss having him to take care of when he is gone.

On a wild and snowy New Year's Eve, two days before Harry's next scheduled transfusion, Miss Pym receives a phone call from the physician.

"Miss Pym? Dr. Chamberlain here. Thank God you're home. I'm at the hospital and I need your help. There's been an awful traffic accident involving a drunk driver and a second car. Two people were killed, but one of the passengers from the second car is still alive. You'll recognize the name. It's Jane Harrison McClintock."

"The peace activist?" Miss Pym can hardly believe what she is hearing.

"That's right. She's in critical condition and I'm not holding out much hope that she'll live, but her chances will improve if we can get some blood into her. The blood bank's run out of reserves on account of the four other accidents we've had to deal with tonight, and the blizzard's put other hospitals right out of the picture. But she's A-negative, so your blood would do just fine. Will you come? Every minute counts now."

"If I come, will I still be able to give blood to Harry on Friday?"

"No—I'm afraid not. We'll need all that's safe to give tonight. It's a terrible choice for you, I know. But with the snow so deep—it'll be days before we're dug out. Miss Pym? Are you there?"

"I'm sorry." Miss Pym's voice comes weakly over the wire. "I'm sorry, Dr. Chamberlain. I wish I could save Miss McClintock. But my brother needs that blood, and if I can only save one person, it will have to be my brother."

This story is our own bioethical variant of "The Archbishop Fenelon," a classic in the ethics literature. The original was conceived two hundred years ago by William Godwin, the father of Mary Wollstonecraft Shelley. Godwin's version, as presented in his *Enquiry Concerning Political Justice* (1793), poses the choice of a man's having to rescue from a fire either the famous writer and cleric Archbishop Fenelon, or Fenelon's valet, who, although comparatively dispensible, happens to be the potential rescuer's own father. Godwin's considered preference in earlier editions of his *Enquiry* was for Fenelon; later, he came to acknowledge that a case, even on the grounds of impartial reason, could be made for saving the father. And indeed, he was right: if the aim of morality is to maximize the happiness of everyone considered impartially, then, given the psychological realities of human life, choosing a low-profile father (or alcoholic brother) over a high-ranking cleric or internationally prominent peace activist isn't obviously immoral. We do, after all, need to trust our intimates to give us special consideration. If we couldn't rely on them in times of trouble, then a deep and pervasive kind of human satisfaction would be lost.

Godwin's change of heart concerning the archbishop has received a fair amount of attention from professional ethicists over the centuries, but recently Bernard Williams put a somewhat different spin on the matter. Suppose a man has read the later edition of Godwin and reflects that he should rescue his wife because (a) she is, after all, his wife, and (b) spouses may show each other some preference in situations where their interests conflict with the interests of nonspouses. Williams wryly notes that such a man has had "a thought too many." If the man justifies his action by appealing to a moral principle that obeys the canons of universalizability and impartiality (*any* spouse may favor a spouse—it has nothing especially to do with these two people), he reveals that something is defective in his love for his wife.[12]

The point here is that the favoritism we show to those we love doesn't derive its moral justification from sources of goodness other than love. Favoritism is part of what it *is* to love, and it takes whatever moral force it has from the value of the love itself. Love, to put it another way, inherently plays favorites.

Further, its value can't be wholly encompassed by impartial principles. Impartial principles would bid us to favor the interests of our loved ones over the interests of others just to the point where we contribute to the overall good and no further. As we admitted earlier, this may seem right, since one concern in developing a moral account of family relationships has got to be finding the limits to favoritism. (Sincere and deep love may justify giving needed blood to your brother rather than to a charismatic peace activist, but it doesn't justify holding down the activist, kicking and screaming, to get bone marrow for your brother.) It becomes evident, however, that wherever the limit on favoritism is placed, it can't be precisely at the threshold where the impartialist moral theorist would place it. If it is really favoritism we are talking about here—and hence real love, rather than some ersatz version—then it must resist, at least to some degree, the pull of others' interests. Otherwise, it is simply disguised impartiality and not real love at all. Like the disguised instrumentality that deluded the broken-hearted opera singer in the last chapter, disguised impartiality isn't capable of conveying the good of love, and ought not to be mistaken for it.

Particularity

Family ethics, like traditional medical ethics (but unlike ethics in general), is importantly situated in the particular and the specific. But the particularities that count for families are, of course, different: not the practices and traditions of a healing profession, but the personalities and life situations of specific family members, as well as common practices or traditions to which families may have allegiance.

Consider a contrast between families and nations. Americans as a nation generally operate on the notion that people should be free to lead their lives as they themselves see fit, providing they obey the law and don't scare the horses; the vision of the good life is deliberately left sketchy, to be filled in by each of us in our own way. In families, on the other hand, the scale is right for people to come to know each other well, and to entertain and pursue a vision of what it is to live well that is richer than that shared by the country at large. That richness is a product of the many little particulars that make up the pattern of daily family life. Like a religious community, or a feminist collective, a family can affirm certain values and repudiate others *en famille*, so that the small details of the daily routine form a mosaic of shared meaning. Contributing to that mosaic of particulars can promote a feeling of solidarity among family members which is in itself a deep source of personal satisfaction.

Particulars play a strong role in self-definition: I am this specific person with this unique history. Families also define themselves through the particular details of their ongoing history, not only by painting their summer cottages or speaking Polish, but by moving in certain moral directions. Accumulated little instances of family hospitality, for example, might allow a certain family to feel it is "in character" to welcome an HIV-infected foster-child into the household. There are important implications in these family histories for medical decisionmaking.

Nonconsensuality

As a culture, our moral self-understanding—or at least our moral rhetoric—is highly influenced by the notions of consent and contract. We sometimes define obligation in terms of consent, even when we have to go to rather contorted lengths to do it.[13] We fail to notice that obligations can arise from other forms of human behavior as well. For example, if I were to smash your Ming vase, I would be under an obligation to make good the loss. Causal relationships like this can produce just as firm obligations as agreements can. It's possible, of course, to give a consent-based account of why I owe you restitution for your vase—I consented to enter your house and therby tacitly agreed to acknowledge liability for any accident that occurred there; there's a contract that governs social interactions in general and that binds me to certain obligations in the matter of broken vases, and so on—but one can always ask why my tacit consent to enter houses or take part in polite society ought to carry a rider to the effect that I'm responsible for damage I cause, unless I'm in fact responsible *because* I caused the damage.

Similarly, we want to suggest, not all obligations incurred inside families are based on contract or consent. Although marriage in contemporary America is indeed entered into by mutual agreement, children notoriously "didn't ask to be born," and none of us choose our blood relations. Yet common morality recognizes duties to parents, siblings, and other relatives. Where do these duties come from? That's a complex question.

Parents' duties to children, we'll argue, arise from their direct responsibility for bringing the children into existence, whether they meant to or not—and for putting them into the world in a condition of such extreme vulnerability that they will die without care. Because they put them into this predicament, it's up to the parents to provide for them until the children are old enough to take care of themselves. Nor can one parent release the other from this responsibility, as it is the child, and not the other parent, to whom the debt is owed. To make this obligation a matter of consent would be to validate abandonment, perpetuating the ancient pattern whereby a man sires a child and then walks away on the grounds that he's not really ready for fatherhood.

As for adult children's duty to care for their ailing parents, we'll suggest that this comes from the relationships the parents were obliged to establish when the children were young. It is up to parents to teach their children how to be social beings, which means, among other things, teaching them how to love. The parents do this by putting themselves into a loving relationship with their children—a relationship which will be one-sided at first, but later, as the child learns how to love back, will become mutual. In establishing this loving intimacy, the parents put themselves in the child's power, and if the child then repudiates the parent in need, the parent's trust in the bond will have been betrayed. We'll expand on these arguments in Chapters Five and Six; here, we merely want to suggest that the idea of freely choosing one's duties can't do all the work that an ethics of the family requires.

This nonconsensual aspect of family life, especially when coupled with the imbalance of power that obtains when young children, the chronically ill, or the frail elderly are dependent on family members with greater prestige, mobility, and resources, can be a major source of oppression, and is perhaps the primary reason why, in the late-twentieth-century climate of ethical individualism, families are so often mistrusted. But if it is true that great suffering comes from mistreatment at the hands of people you are not free to leave, it is also true that if you are always free to leave you can't get the good of settled, abiding relationships. Indeed, even where we choose our intimates freely, once the choice is made we are not free to leave at will, because intimacy changes the very identities of the persons involved, so that to destroy the relationship is to damage the selves within it. Sometimes this becomes necessary, but the person doing it must have a very good reason.

To acknowledge the nonconsensual element in families and in other settings of intimacy is not to deny that there are general (universalizable, impartial) moral constraints that operate within them as well. The disturbing prevalence of abuse within intimate contexts is clearly wrong; it outrages our general moral sense, and any account of morality that doesn't roundly condemn the ill-usage of helpless people should be tossed out on those grounds alone. But the abuse of intimates takes on a special wrongfulness in part because of the moral features of intimate living that are *not* well represented by general accounts. Abuse of an intimate ruptures trust in a very deep and damaging way, and studies indicate that the survivors of such abuse tend to suffer more deeply than do those who have been abused by strangers.[14]

The special wrongfulness of the abuse of intimates backlights, as it were, the special moral significance of intimate relationships.

NO PART OF HIS LIFE PLAN

Philip and his cousin George grew up together in an Irish neighborhood in South Buffalo. Philip's dad was a dockworker, and on certain Saturday mornings he used to take the little boys to see the Great Lakes freighters offload their cargoes. The boys were almost daily playmates who quarreled and fought, invented games and explored the neighborhood with great amity. When Philip was six and George a year younger, George's widowed mother died and her children were fostered out to various relatives. George came to live with Philip's family and was adopted by them soon after.

The boys had very different temperaments, but perhaps on account of this they remained close friends. Philip played a terrific game of sandlot baseball; George merely collected baseball cards. Philip never developed the habit of reading; George read aloud to him in bed at night after their light was supposed to be out. In high school they ran with the same crowd and on occasion they even dated the same girls. When Philip was married, George stood best man. When George was divorced, Philip took him to the tavern to drown his sorrow.

Philip put together a nice life for himself. He began as a carpenter, but through hard work soon developed a flourishing business as a building contractor. By the time he was thirty-five he and his wife and kids lived in a two-story colonial in Amherst.

George wasn't so lucky. He made it through college and became a schoolteacher, mostly seventh and eighth grade English, but shortly after his marriage collapsed he noticed he had become clumsier than usual—he was dropping things and fumbling when he tried to tie his shoes. A series of tests confirmed what the physician already suspected: he had amyotrophic lateral sclerosis, sometimes called Lou Gehrig's disease, which would leave him progressively debilitated until, in a few years at best, he would be completely paralyzed.

His health insurance was all right, but at some point he would have to give up his job and he'd then no longer be able to live alone. He turned to Philip, but Philip declined to help. A coolness sprang up between them and within a year all contact had been broken. Philip was fond enough of his cousin, but, as he told his wife privately, it was no part of his life plan to look after someone who was dying a slow death.

In nonintimate contexts—in business, court, or school—we can claim the same kind of moral respect that anyone else gets; we can expect that our rights will be honored and our dignity observed. But in intimate contexts we are owed much more: love and importance, fidelity and solidarity, all grounded in the fine-grained particulars of lives lived in common. That's why Philip's behavior may strike us as sleazy. It's not merely that he's being selfish; it's that he's betrayed the years of intimacy and trust that give George a moral claim on his care.

Premodern Sensibility

Finally, families are grounded in ancient, even archaic values that have been overlain with more modern conceptions of right behavior. Such values are the social equivalent of the gingko tree, which flourished in the time of the dinosaurs but also does fairly well amid the exhaust fumes of the contemporary city. The ancient moral character of families can be seen in the institution of hereditary monarchy and the testamentary disposition of property, in the special duties parents owe their children and children their parents, and in the special claims that our kin often have on our time, money, and attention. Because the institution of the family is so very old, we can expect it to display vestiges of earlier world views, much as the English language contains archaic word-formations and grammatical constructions, or the city of Rome shelters a variety of ancient architectural styles. Much of the tension families experience when they encounter the health care system comes from these vestiges of the family's moral past.

The general, medical, and familial ethics surveyed here share a set of similar functions despite their differences: by guiding each of us toward admirable action and habits of discernment and integrity, they enhance our own characters and ease our lives together. However, the ways in which the ethics of families does diverge from both general ethics and other "local" ethics like those of medicine can bring confusion. At worst, this divergence distorts both medicine and families, and troubles the harmony of their relationship. The threat of confusion, distortion, and disharmony calls for political response: negotiation, the construction of new structures for living together, the passage of new laws, the development of professions. It also calls for individual response: accepting new ideals, situating them coherently within the constellation of our persisting goals, developing new virtues. To get anywhere with this restructuring of medicine, families, and ourselves, we're going to have to see clearly and vividly what we're aiming for. We need something to light our way.

Stars to Steer By

A long-standing dream of our culture has been to develop a system of ethics around a single, central value, or, at least, to rank-order distinct values in a strict and clear way. The great attraction of this vision is that the task of living well within oneself and with others is simplified if every choice can be assessed according to how it chimes in with what's fundamentally important.

This yearning is expressed in Plato's account of "The Form of the Good." To Plato's way of thinking, what's truly worthy of admiration and pursuit has an objective nature, which can be perceived by an appropriately prepared person who can then rule herself or a Republic with real justice. The power of this vision hasn't altogether faded; the great systems of Mill and Kant, which exert so much force on our contemporary accounts of medical ethics, are both attempts to achieve such unified versions of morality.

Unfortunately, reducing everything we value to some common denominator like "the good" or "utility," or "the categorical imperative" seems increasingly less likely to succeed. In fact, as these well-known moral theories begin to lose their grip on the academic understanding of common morality—a process that has received considerable help from feminists, postmodern thinkers, and even philosophers who are closely associated with the mainstream of their profession—we encounter and take seriously forms of value that have been muted by the passion to develop a unified, simple system of ethics.[15] The values of intimacy, with their focus on the personal and the particular, are a prime example.

But if all the things we value can't be seen as instances of some one master value, or neatly ranked in one Great Chain of Being, then moral life becomes much less a matter of calculation and more a matter of navigation, of trying to steer a prudent course among independent and sometimes incompatible values. We must neither ignore any of these values, nor allow ourselves to be overmastered by any of them; either way lies ruin. What we now must do is to distill some of these general ideas about the special moral significance of families into navigational aids—"stars to steer by," as it were—so as to help family members chart a safe passage among the rocks and shoals of contemporary medical practice. At the same time, these stars should also help physicians, other health care workers, and family members themselves see the value of families properly. By their light, they should be able to avoid seeing the flaws of families too cynically and their virtues too romantically.

Throughout the rest of this book, we will be using these stars to light the ethical landscape. They are intended, not so much as rules for conduct, or even as facts that override other considerations, but as reminders of why we need to shift our understanding of the two systems of care under consideration. We will invoke these stars as we consider questions like why reigning views of medicine lose sight of families. We hope to use the stars to guide us to a new orientation, whereby the two systems honor and help each other. The stars are these:

* *Family Members Aren't Replaceable by Similarly (or Better) Qualified People*
* *Family Members Are Stuck with Each Other*
* *The Need for Intimacy Produces Responsibilities*
* *Causing Someone to Exist Produces Responsibilities*
* *Virtues Are Learned at Our Mother's (and Father's) Knees*
* *Families Are Ongoing Stories*
* *In Families, Motives Matter a Lot*

Each of these stars deserves a closer look.

Family Members Aren't Replaceable by Similarly (or Better) Qualified People

Most social systems we encounter regard the individuals who make them up as interchangeable, to one degree or another. This is because the most important ends served by such systems are external: the point of a hospital is not to enhance the lives of its employees, but to respond to the illness and injury of patients; the point of a school is not to foster caring relationships among its staff, but to educate its students. That's why hospital employees, school staff, farm workers, or people in any other occupation are to a certain extent replaceable by others similarly or better qualified. The organizations they populate are identified by the roles those people occupy, and the ends the organizations serve are distinguishable from the personal ends of those people.

Surely a decent hospital, school, or farm will treat its workers with respect, and try to foster in them a sense of belonging and of personal investment in the aims and character of the institution. But to a significant degree their motivation for treating workers well is instrumental: well-treated employees are much more likely to serve the institution efficiently. You can't run a good organization by discharging someone whenever anybody better comes along, but the fact remains that workers are chosen in large part for their qualifications. If they expect to keep their jobs they have to exercise these qualifications properly.

Families don't work like that, because their fundamental point is not to serve an external end. This isn't to say that families don't serve such ends—they socialize and nurture the young, they provide emotional comfort and sources of identity and identification for us all—but these tasks aren't what families are ultimately about. Rather, their function is to cherish individual members, not for contributions to various ends, but for themselves.

Families, of course, aren't static; clearly, people do get "discharged" and "replaced" in them through divorce and remarriage, through death and birth. But the stories behind such changes, and their effects upon the family and its identity as a whole, are much deeper and more profound than those that characterize personnel shifts in other organizations.

Family Members Are Stuck with Each Other

This star keeps close company with the first. With the complex exceptions of marriage, marriagelike commitments, and adoption, we don't choose familial relations, we don't replace family members with other, better qualified people, and we can't just walk away from these relationships if the fancy strikes us. By and large, then, we are "stuck" each other, and that means that we are stuck with certain claims on our attention, resources, and behavior. To be someone's parent, child, sibling, or cousin is to be in a relationship founded in biology and history, not in contractual conventions. An individual's decision can no more dissolve such relationships than it can negate any other historical fact.

To acknowledge this is not to deny that what we make of the situation is largely up to us; one can imagine forms of human life in which it matters hardly at all. But as a matter of fact, we *have* made a great deal of it. As a matter of biology and history, occupying family roles intersects with a variety of considerations we regard as morally important. There is a rich set of expectations that we associate with such roles, and we're particularly vulnerable to deep disappointment and even damage if those expectations are simply shrugged off. Indeed, as we press harder at why we have those expectations, and at the nature of our disappointment if they aren't fulfilled, we find the expectations themselves are based on other deeply held beliefs about human life. As our first star reminds us, seeing families as composed of replaceable parts is inconsistent with our understanding of what an intimate relationship is, and with the ability of such relationships to convey the special goods of intimacy. Also, certain familial roles reflect deeply held beliefs about how responsibilities are acquired and discharged.

It may not be clear, as the nineteenth-century philosopher Henry Sidgwick wrote, what a child owes a parent; what a child owes siblings or more loosely connected relatives is even less clear.[16] But it is clear that close biological kinship overlaps with social and personal patterns of meaning and moral relation, so much so that simply dismissing one's parents or siblings or the cousin one was reared with seems wrong. Moral relationships among family members can certainly be strained by betrayal or violence, but it takes a catastrophe to dissolve them; they can't be set aside merely as a matter of inclination or decision. To the extent that we are so closely entwined in the life of another that we become an important part of that person, we truly are stuck with each other.

The Need for Intimacy Produces Responsibilities

Intimacy is a complex force, and not uniformly positive. Intimate relationships typically involve relaxing the defenses we wind about ourselves, to shield us from others and to simplify our interactions with them. Because our guard is down, such relationships create vulnerability. At the same time, they give us the opportunity to know ourselves more fully; they give us chances to know and feel the richness of other people, to acknowledge concretely and vividly that they matter.

The benefits of intimate relationships come with the responsibility not to abuse the special confidence placed in us. Intimates can not only hurt each other's feelings, but also impede each others' ability to enter more deeply into intimacy. While something similar could be said for nonintimate relationships (the liar erodes not only trust in her own word, but, to some extent, trust in language itself), the significance and particularity of intimacy make this threat especially serious.

Just as intimate relationships themselves aren't always the result of "free choice," so the responsibilities that stem from them are often not freely chosen. Part of what we do in such relationships is precisely to bind each other with particular, unchosen responsibilities. This raises the question of just what obligations we have no choice but to accept, and what responses to others go above and beyond the call of duty. Fine-grained answers to these questions are developed in the ensuing chapters; however, as a preliminary account, it seems to us that the general form of intimate responsibility must be to guard intimates in those areas where the relationship itself leaves them vulnerable.

Causing Someone to Exist Produces Responsibilities

This aspect of family life continues the theme of noncontractual duties and relationships. The character of family goals and the nature of intimacy will often generate obligations one never agreed to, as we have said above and as any teenager will tell you; the fact that families are also settings in which new people come into the world adds another noncontractual element to the picture. To return to our earlier example, if I bring a child into the world, I cause a morally considerable person to undergo severe risk of harm: the baby will die unless it is cared for. The fact that I caused the baby's predicament means I have a responsibility to try to avert the harm that threatens it. Even if I've been forced or tricked into becoming a parent, I still owe this to the child even if I do it by finding acceptable substitute parents. As we will see later, this observation is particularly useful as we try to make sense of who counts as a parent in contract pregnancy and in the various other forms of assisted reproduction that medical technology has made possible.

Virtues Are Learned at Our Mother's (and Father's) Knee

Families serve as our first and perhaps most fundamental school for moral formation; this description is trotted out so often that it has become a platitude. And so it invites the standard reaction to platitudes: we tend to think it's either trivial or false. The fact that high school commencement speakers and presidential candidates keep pointing out the major significance of the family's role in moral formation, though, is no reason to disbelieve it.

Families are an excellent place for foundational work in morals, and not only because children are impressionable and parents can hector them about "right" behavior. The more fundamental reason is that it is there that children learn how to live within the set of relationships in which they're nested.

Any kind of advanced education in ethics—learning ethical theory, for example, with a view to applying it to the practice of medicine—presupposes a great deal of such early training. A desire to do the right thing, even when it involves a certain amount of personal cost, underscores all analyses of tough cases or difficult issues, and it has to be instilled as a habit. Reading great literature, studying moral theory, or even contemplating the lives of the saints isn't very likely to have much of an influence on one's character unless virtuous habits have been laid down early on.

The parallels between the family as linguistic community and the family as moral community are instructive. Just as (most) children are born with the ability to generate very complex grammatical structures, which they do with astonishing speed as they begin to manipulate their linguistic environment, so too do they enter the world with the emotions and the cognitive capacity necessary to form a complex value structure, which is then played out in imitation of those around them.

Precisely how this works is a complicated question, but what seems clear is that the old romantic notion of the child as *tabula rasa*—a blank slate to be written upon by parents or corrupting social forces—is as mistaken as the idea that children enter the world with vicious dispositions that require continual parental vigilance to correct. Rather, current psychological opinion converges on the idea that moral emotions, present at birth, motivate the acquisition of virtues, which are fostered within the relationships the child is born into or forges as she grows older. Jerome Kagan has identified five candidates for the emotional states that form the basis of morality: (1) anticipation of anxiety in response to physical harm, social disapproval, or failure to perform a task; (2) the feeling of empathy toward those who are in need or at risk; (3) the feeling of responsibility following recognition that one has caused distress or harm to another; (4) the feeling of ennui or fatigue following repeated gratifications of a desire; (5) the feeling of uncertainty accompanying events one doesn't understand or inconsistency between one's beliefs and one's actions.[17] Kagan notes that people don't like to feel afraid, to feel sorry for others in need, or to feel guilty, bored, or confused, and so, he thinks, they are motivated to dispositions and actions that avoid these feelings, in the idiom of the culture to which they are born. For example, the four virtues of fifth-century Athens—courage, justice, wisdom, and prudence—might in nineteenth-century Boston become loyalty to personal convictions, charity toward the poor, insight into one's intentions, and moderation of ambition. Kagan points out that Peter Geach's candidates for virtue also fit this schemata: faith and hope allay the depression and apathy that follow recognition that a desired goal is unattainable; charity mutes sympathetically induced disquiet; and prudence shields us from worry over possible loss of wealth and reputation.

Both Kagan's and Geach's way of putting the matter strike us as unnecessarily dark, however. Surely pleasurable as well as painful feelings serve as the basis for morality; human beings are just as motivated by a desire to please as by fear of displeasure, and Hume's notion of sympathy is the sunnier version of Kagan's empathy. But the general idea seems plausible enough: we are born with prosocial feelings that motivate our behavior toward others, and our first forays into distributive justice, caring for others, and standing up for what is right even in the face of opposition are guided by our parents and take place among siblings or playmates.[18]

Indeed, children without siblings are at a disadvantage when it comes to moral development. Psychologists in mainland China, curious about the effect on children of the centralized State Family Planning Commission's implementation of the one-child family policy, recently studied a thousand kindergarten and elementary school children, comparing those with siblings to those without on a range of social and cognitive dimensions. They found that children with no brothers or sisters were more self-centered, acting more in accord with their own interests and cooperating less with others; they were less well liked by the other children and less able to cope with constraints and frustrations. A family environment with siblings, the researchers concluded, is an important part of a child's moral upbringing.[19]

Families are also crucial to the formation of a child's conscience. If conscience is understood as "the exercise and expression of a reflective sense of integrity," as "the voice of one's self as a whole," which integrates personal history, reason, emotion, imagination, and action, then insofar as the family gives a child its sense of self (as we argued in Chapter Two that it does), it gives the child the stuff of conscience.[20] The Freudian idea that we internalize familial socialization can't account for the normative force of appeals to conscience—we don't follow the claims of conscience because they mirror the family's values but because we sincerely and on critical reflection believe them to be correct. It is certainly possible to follow the voice of conscience and do wrong, but to whatever extent our families play a role in making us who we are, they influence this voice of one's self, whose demands on us are stringent indeed.

So, a disposition toward morality is part of the legacy of early experience, at least for those favored enough to enjoy some stability, some care, and someone to care for. If the child is even more fortunate, it will be reared in a family that provides motivation and direction to see morality as an undertaking that lends a special character to life, that imparts to life a significance that can outlast a person's own life and own concerns.

Families Are Ongoing Stories

Much of what happens at any given moment in families takes its significance from what has gone before and will go behind. Families are often sites whose significance is both "dense" and "extended": much of what goes on takes place inside a configuration of persons and events that pulls together richly developed themes extending across generations. This feature of families is itself a source of moral guidance, as children learn from the family "stories" that extend into the past. When questions about the future suggest themselves, family decisionmakers are faced with the issue of how that legacy can and should guide them, even as they continue its story in the present and into the future.

There's a natural temptation for each individual in the family to suppose she is the sole author of her own story. But in families, stories are coauthored. A family may have the kind of plot outline whereby Mother's expression of anger is perceived as far less disturbing to everybody than an angry expression very similar in occasion, volume, and content from Father. This sort of thing can be annoying to Father—after all, we want to be understood as meaning just what we do mean by our actions and words, and no more or less. But meaning isn't simply a private matter, a "word balloon" that anyone can place on anything he says or does independently of the background text. Neither is that backdrop immutable, and in many instances it ought to be rewritten so that those acting in front of it can go in a substantially new direction as time goes on. But this narrative background is too important to ignore, and its potential usefulness as a way of understanding and resolving moral problems can be of considerable value.

In Families, Motives Matter a Lot

Our view of people's motives, intentions, and mental states can transform our assessment of them and their deeds. An altered picture of a deed's motivation can turn mistakes (forgetting to pay a debt) into crimes (withholding money on purpose), or transform assault and battery (thrusting a knife into someone) into health care (surgery). Even between strangers it matters whether a transaction is conducted with respect or contempt, out of friendliness or irritation: remember how you felt the last time a grocery-store clerk made it clear that ringing up your produce was a serious inconvenience?

But if motives matter among strangers, among intimates they take on an added significance. In his discussion in the *Nicomachean Ethics* on the duties grown children owe their aged parents, Aristotle argues that among intimates intention is everything. What counts is that children try to befriend their parents, and it is their intention rather than their success or failure that shows whether they are doing their best, "for it is purpose that is the characteristic thing in a friend and in virtue." (1164b2)

It seems that the most natural way of understanding how difference in purpose can alter the moral quality of an act is to focus on what the action "conveys" or "expresses."[21] The same action done from different motives does have a different expressive quality: think again of the broken-hearted opera singer, whose wife encouraged him, not because she loved him, but to enhance his self-esteem enough so that she could leave him. Motives are crucial where the goal is to care for someone, and hence, motivation is important in medicine. But it is even more important in settings where care is richer, deeper, and more personal, as in many families.

In families, actions motivated by duty, or by concern for what others may think, are less significant than the same actions motivated by love. The reason is that certain motivations are themselves a tangible good of intimacy, conveyed piggyback on whatever other good the action contains. You don't look for love from a nurse who massages your skin to prevent bedsores, but when the masseuse is your own daughter, the backrub means something different.

In the four chapters to follow we will use our seven stars in an attempt to work out concretely and in detail resolutions to some of the conflicts of value that are so damaging both to medicine and to families. The stars will serve, again, not as moral rules or even guides for conduct, but as reminders of the morally peculiar nature of the institution of the family as it comes into contact with medicine in four broad areas: making treatment decisions, caring for the frail elderly, seeking reproductive help, and setting appropriate limits on care.

Chapter Four

Medical Decisionmaking

DECISIONMAKING HAS BEEN THE MAJOR AREA OF CONTINUED ETHICAL interest in medicine. Indeed, it's not too much to claim that the bioethical revolution of the last twenty years has largely consisted of a shift in the way medical decisions are made in the United States: where once the physician, acting on the principle of beneficence, decided what was best for the patient, such behavior is now considered paternalistic and unethical, because it fails to respect the patient's right to decide these matters for himself.

As long ago as 1914 the noted jurist Benjamin Cardozo affirmed this right in the case of *Schloendorff v. Society of New York Hospital.* In *Schloendorff,* a physician removed a fibroid tumor after a patient had consented to abdominal exploration under anesthesia, but had explicitly ruled out surgery. Judge Cardozo proclaimed that a "human being of adult years and sound mind" has a "right to determine what shall be done with his body."[1] But determining the exact meaning of this credo, applying it to particular cases, weighing the legitimacy of social encroachments on it, and building up a consensus regarding its correctness both within the medical community and outside it has been an ongoing process that will doubtless continue for some time yet. There is now general agreement that the patient's consent is required for treatment, and that it's the physician's duty to inform the patient so that the consent isn't coerced through manipulation of the patient's ignorance of medicine. Further, it's the physician's duty to understand that not all the values that enter the decisionmaking process are medical values. More important for the patient might be personal values that have little to do with mere bodily health but everything to do with the patient's conception of a good life—something the physician is in no position to dictate. For this reason, the process of informed consent has to embrace the notion of informed refusal, which the physician must respect even when she disagrees with the patient.[2]

This shift in the ethics of decisionmaking has forced the medical profession to redefine its goals. The ends of medicine are less frequently taken to be purely and simply saving life and restoring physical and mental functioning, or, where cure is impossible, doing what can be done to ease suffering. These are still central, but now they are embedded in a process of setting goals that are consistent with what's important to the patient as well as the professional integrity of the physician.[3] Where the patient is too ill to let others know what's important to him, it's still considered a necessary part of good medical practice to determine as best one can what he would have requested, were he able to speak for himself. In fact, this trend has gathered such momentum that some ethicists speak of the need to anticipate what a patient *would want*, even if the patient is a baby who is too young to have any coherent sense of what it personally considers important.

So decisionmaking is a messier business than it used to be, not only because the patient's wishes must be considered, but also because biotechnology keeps producing more and more medical options. Bioethics has had a lot to say about all this, pitching its advice mostly to physicians but also to nurses (seldom to patients). Bioethicists have, however, largely been silent about the moral significance of the family in medical decisionmaking.

The third edition of the bioethical bible, Beauchamp and Childress's *Principles of Biomedical Ethics*, discusses the family explicitly in only one paragraph, stating that the burden on the family shouldn't be the decisive factor in decisions to withhold treatment from a patient.[4] Another book of major significance, *Deciding to Forego Life-Sustaining Treatment*, authored by the President's Commission for the Study of Ethical Problems in Medicine and Biomedical and Behavioral Research, devotes no more than ten lines of text in 545 pages to the family's role in helping patients make and implement decisions at the end of life. Alan Buchanan and Dan Brock's influential *Deciding for Others* expends much of its brief discussion of the family on the possibility of selfishness and disagreement among family members. The Hastings Center's equally influential *Guidelines on the Termination of Life-Sustaining Treatment and the Care of the Dying* mentions families only in passing, in their role as surrogate decisionmakers or as people who have feelings for the patient.

Why the neglect? Because, we submit, the value of families, while often nodded to, is typically misunderstood. They are seen as nothing more than collections of individuals, each seeking to maximize his own self-interest. While Buchanan and Brock, for example, point out that "the family as an intimate association is one important way in which individuals find or construct meaning in their lives," they immediately go on to discuss mechanisms for safeguarding the patient from being exploited by his next of kin. They explain that it's all right to permit families, rather than physicians or the courts, to be surrogate decisionmakers for those too young or ill to decide for themselves, because "the context in which the more serious medical treatment or care decisions are usually made typically provides significant safeguards to inhibit decisions that promote the family's interest at the expense of the incompetent person's welfare." They then specify a number of conditions that require the hospital or nursing home to intervene in the family's decisionmaking process—conditions ranging from evidence of familial abuse of the patient, to cases in which the patient is particularly vulnerable to harm, to any decision for treatment (as opposed to nontreatment) which, in the view of the physician, is not "medically sound."[5]

While prudence is always appropriate in considering how one person should decide for another, there is an air of distrust running through all this which sits uneasily with Buchanan and Brock's acknowledgment of the significance of families in our lives. Some of this tension, at least, is due to their unwillingness to impute any moral significance to such notions as family solidarity or collective responsibility. Despite their use of the term "the family's interest" in the passage we just cited, they deny that this is anything but shorthand for the interests of *individuals* within the family:

> To speak of the family as having its own goals and purposes and to speak of the familial perspective and familial objectives is to engage in dangerous reification. . . . Talk about group interests is in general warranted only under two circumstances, neither of which obtains in the case at hand: (1) The group has expressed some preference through a collective decision-making process (e.g., voting) or (2) there is something that is in the interest of all members of the group individually. (pp. 236–37)

If you think that only individual people can have goals, purposes, and interests then what Brock and Buchanan have to say here sounds reasonable enough. In point of fact, however, it's not only individuals, but all kinds of things, from the simplest artifact to the most complex multinational corporation, that can have goals and purposes, and these can be quite distinct from the goals of those making up or using the thing in question. For example, you might use your wine bottle exclusively as a rolling-pin, but there is still a correct answer to the question, "What is this for?" which refers to holding wine, and which is based in the bottle's design. A basketball team has winning as its goal, even if some of its members have accepted bribes to throw games; striving to win is part of the design of competitive sports, and this design can't be altogether reduced to the interests of the athletes on a given squad.

Families, too, have purposes which, like winning a competition, can only be accomplished through the activities of individuals, but which are not reducible to individual desires or attitudes; there are some things, as it were, that families are for, and we may quite properly regard as being "in their interests" the circumstances and conditions that are conducive to achieving those ends. Once we recognize this, we'll be prepared to see that all the conflicts that may go on within families aren't necessarily conflicts between individuals or subgroups of individuals: some will be clashes between what an individual family member needs or wants, and the things a family needs so it can do its special job of conveying the goods of intimacy.

Substituted Judgment

The legal justification for turning to families for decisions about treatment for patients who are incapable of making their own is, first, that an incompetent patient's right to refuse medical care can be exercised through a proxy.[6] Second, as the family knows the patient's wishes well, it can "make the decision that the incompetent patient would make if he or she were competent."[7] To the extent that the proxy can stand in the patient's shoes, choosing the same course of action under the circumstances that the patient would, the proxy exercises *substituted judgment* on behalf of the patient.

The New Jersey Supreme Court summed up this approach rather nicely in its 1987 ruling in the case of Nancy Ellen Jobes. Pregnant when involved in an automobile accident, Ms. Jobes had suffered irreversible brain damage in the course of an operation to remove her dead fetus. The New Jersey court wrote:

> When an irreversibly vegetative patient like Mrs. Jobes has not clearly expressed her intentions with respect to medical treatment, the *Quinlan* "substituted judgment" approach best accomplishes the goal of having the patient make her own decision. In most cases in which the "substituted judgment" doctrine is applied, the surrogate decisionmaker will be a family member or close friend of the patient. Generally it is the patient's family or other loved ones who support and care for the patient, and who best understand the patient's personal values and beliefs. Hence they will be best able to make a substituted judgment for the patient.[8]

Again, this is the sort of claim that at first seems to make perfect sense. The trouble is, the notion that the family best understands the patient's personal values and beliefs doesn't stand up to careful examination. Good, hard empirical data are accumulating to the effect that, when people are asked to predict what medical treatment a member of the family would want under a variety of scenarios if the person were to become incompetent, they get it wrong about half the time: flipping a coin would be almost as accurate.[9] There seems to be good agreement between patients and proxies about what kind of medical treatment the competent patient would currently want, but when asked to suppose that these decisions are being made in the aftermath of a stroke or when the patient is demented—that is, in just the kind of situations that would make proxy decisionmaking necessary—this agreement falls off sharply.

We shouldn't be surprised by this. If we stop to think about it, we can see that there's a tremendous imaginative effort involved in synthesizing what one knows about a person's past practices, gestures, decisions, statements, and beliefs so that one can construct that person's response to a new and very specific set of circumstances. There's no direct deductive relationship between general values and a particular set of choices, or between a previous opinion and a present one, particularly when a number of general values are set into conflict. Often, the most one can hope for is creative guesswork on the part of the proxy, who, if she or he is distraught over the patient's condition or worn down by months or years of care and worry, may not be capable of achieving the state of fine awareness and rich responsivity that is required for a successful act of the imagination.

Furthermore, as Patricia D. White has pointed out, the person whose choice the proxy is trying to predict often doesn't know what she herself would want. White, who in the course of her legal practice is often consulted as an estate planner, has had frequent occasion to observe the uncertainty and indecision her clients experience when they try to imagine *themselves* ill and incompetent. They often don't know how to think about it, or even how to think about the "rather different sorts of situations in which a person might find himself needing a proxy medical decision maker."[10] This too seems perfectly natural; when confronted with a novel situation, one can't always guarantee one's response. Consider a woman, pregnant for the first time and convinced that natural childbirth is best for both her and the baby, who in labor changes her mind and asks for pain control. She very likely surprised herself—but then, she's never given birth before.

Best Interests

Difficulties of this kind, along with the perplexities raised when the patient in question is a baby or is severely mentally retarded and so was never able to form wishes or make them known, have led some to recommend that families use a "best interests" standard as a kind of default mode.[11] Under this standard, the decisionmaker is supposed to weigh the benefits and burdens of the various treatment options in the light of the patient's prognosis and current state of suffering, and choose the treatment that seems likeliest to advance the patient's most important interests. Advancing all the patient's interests at once will likely be impossible, and it is also necessary to avoid choices that tax the body more than they heal it. The idea, then, is to opt for the course of action with the greatest net benefit to the patient.[12] Because much of this assessment requires clinical expertise, the physician and ethicist Linda Emanuel has suggested that "identifying the patient's best interests should often be left to the physician."[13]

The problem with this suggestion is that the intricate calculus of burdens and benefits dictated by the "best interests" standard is glaringly incomplete without a judgment of the quality of the patient's present state of life. This is not solely a medical judgment, and no physician can claim special expertise in making it. It is, in fact, a judgment no reflective person should be eager to make, as it seems perilously close to the *lebenswertes Leben* judgments the Nazis employed to justify extermination of the mentally and physically disabled. It is wrong, for example, to allow someone who is demented and incontinent to die of an easily treatable illness on the grounds that life under those conditions isn't worth living. But we can make a distinction here. We can hold firmly to the belief that all persons, no matter what the quality of their life, are to be valued and respected, but at the same time we can make a judgment about what a person's life is worth *to that person*—whether she herself would judge her present life worth living, or no different from being dead, or worse than no further life at all. The question then is not, "Should people who are demented and diapered be allowed to live?" nor even, "Would I, college-educated and clever, and personally fastidious, want to prolong my life if I were demented and diapered?" but, Does *this woman, as she is now,* experience something good when her hair is brushed or when she sits in the sunlight, when she tastes split-pea soup or feels the caress of a nurse's hand—and is this of sufficient value to her to count as a reason to go on?[14]

Even if the quality-of-life objection can be overcome, "best interests" is a tough standard. It is most often used in adversarial situations, such as child custody cases, where there is reason to distrust the motives or the clearheadedness of the parties to the dispute, or where relationships have broken down to such a degree that people may be forgiven for looking out only for themselves (or the courts forgiven for supposing they should.) The standard works well in situations where people are pitted against each other because it's premised on a view of human nature whose governing principle is that each should do the best for himself that he can. That principle, when people are in competition with one another, is a rational one. While not denying that decisions about the care of an incompetent patient can sometimes take on adversarial proportions, or that occasionally proxy decisionmakers are up to no good, we have seen no data to warrant the belief that decisionmaking for incompetent patients generally takes place in an atmosphere of such mistrust and suspicion that the "best interests" standard is required as a safeguard.

Getting the best for yourself that you can is no part of the morality of families. In families, people have to share their resources (which are usually limited) and while these may not be divided equitably, the idea is that others must be considered. Because family members are bound together in a complex web of love and obligation, life-projects and traditions—a web valued for itself as something that makes life good—a family member will often find it rational *not* to appropriate the best for himself, but to take turns with the others. Someone, now incompetent, who has hewed to this code of conduct all her life might well have wanted to forgo treatment that maximally advances her interests if it is gotten at great emotional or financial cost to the rest of her family. While the "best interest" standard is intended to be invoked only in cases where this sort of thing can't be known, it's still worth bearing in mind that the people upon whom the standard is practiced might have been highly distressed by it.

Besides, it's difficult to take "best interests" literally. If we did, any time a baby was born its parents would have a duty to find the wealthiest, best educated, kindest, highest-principled people they could to rear the child in their stead. A lover would be duty-bound to find the person with whom the beloved could be happiest of all—and then bow out. Doing this would, of course, not be in the best interests of the parents or the lover, so, if *their* interests are also to be maximized, we arrive once again at the each-do-the-best-for-himself-that-he-can principle that characterizes, not families, but something more like the stock market.

Community Standards

Because the "substituted judgment" and "best interests" standard are each problematic in their own way (including one way we haven't even mentioned yet), Linda and Ezekiel Emanuel have recently proposed a third possibility: community standards, hammered out through democratic processes.[15]

They point out that, as vast and pluralistic as the United States is, it will be impossible to get a national consensus on treatment decisions for incapacitated patients that is detailed enough to be practicable; the communities in consensus will have to be smaller, local ones. In some of these, the standards will be "simple procedural standards, such as the adoption of the *Jobes* guidelines, which recognize the family as the de facto decision maker even without proxy forms or other documentation of the patient's wishes."[16] But in other communities certain decisions might simply be prohibited. A community might agree, for example, that people who are permanently comatose ought not to be kept on ventilators, so these patients would simply not be candidates for such treatment, regardless of what their families want.

The proposal is an important and interesting one, because it makes good use of the insight that much of ethics is grounded in the values of the community. It's a more broadly applicable standard of decisionmaking than "substituted judgment" or "best interests of the patient," because it's not only the standard for deciding whether those standards will be used, but also provides explicit guidance on the difficult issue of how a community's interests—in, say, the fair and efficient allocation of scarce resources—should bear on individual treatment decisions.

In addition, the notion of community standards is sufficiently flexible so it can solve the difficulties we encountered with the "substituted judgment" and "best interest" standards. That is, if the community has a rich enough agreement about what human life and death and the goals of medicine are all about, it doesn't matter that proxies aren't terribly accurate at figuring out what a patient would want, because the patient, as a member of the community, can be presumed to share in its opinions. As for best interests, it's all right to let the physician do the fine-grained assessment of not only medical benefits and costs but of the quality of the patient's life, as the physician is presumed to share the community's values, just as the patient does.

There are problems here, though; there are bound to be in a proposal that is still being worked out. One is discussed in Ezekiel Emanuel's *The Ends of Human Life*, where he makes it clear that by "community," he means a sufficiently wide array of community health programs (CHPs) to accommodate the country's cultural pluralism (pp. 178-85). Within each CHP, a democratic process of deliberation would articulate the group's vision of the good life and establish policies for health care, which would be subject to continuous review. Each CHP would have to be highly specific in its view of the good life if it is to make the value judgments required when deciding for others, but a CHP serving only lesbians, to use Emanuel's example, won't do. Such a CHP might get agreement on the legitimacy of a certain sexual orientation, but would very likely run a wide gamut on nearly everything else, embracing communitarians and liberals; radical-separatist feminists, feminists who feel deeply bound to their sons, brothers, and fathers, and women who don't particularly think of themselves as feminists at all; devout, practicing Jews and secular skeptics. Unless your CHP becomes very exclusionary indeed, the thickly shared values needed for achieving consensus about treatment decisions simply won't exist.

Besides, once you have balkanized the country by breaking it up into camps in this way, you are left with the problem of how to negotiate relations among the communities. They would, after all, be embedded within the larger society. Even if you imagine, as Emanuel does, that the communities will all recognize certain basic rights, necessary for the democratic deliberation that is central to the proposal, you have to explain where those rights come from, as they are not obviously derived from the community. You also have to explain how excluding certain people from the community on the basis of their beliefs, race, national origin, or religion is compatible with the values embodied in the Constitution and the Bill of Rights. Further, the wider society would have to be hospitable to the proposal, as "community-based decisions about the termination of care cannot be implemented in isolation but necessitate the creation of more general political and health care reforms."[17] If the United States is too big a community to count as one for present purposes, CHPs would seem to be too small.

Who Will Stand for Me?

In any case, there is a further problem here—the one we said we would describe. In the Emanuels' account, authority to decide for the incompetent, whether delegated to family or friends or kept for itself, comes from the community (probably understood more broadly than the CHP). They reason this way: the only way a person can legitimately be said to exercise agency *for* someone else (as opposed to exercising agency *over* someone else) is if that person knows what the other person would want. Families have been presumed to know this, but studies now indicate that they don't. They cannot, then, perform "substituted judgment," and if they have to fall back on the "best interest" standard because they don't know what the patient would want, they no longer have the right to speak for the patient.[18]

In the absence of special knowledge, the authority of the proxy becomes authority *over* the patient, which must be justified on other grounds than the one of knowledge. What those other grounds might be is a matter for the community to decide, just as it decides about public education, or zoning ordinances, or other details of orderly community life.

But let's look again at the Emanuels' first assumption. Does a proxy's authority rest solely on the proxy's knowledge of how the other person would decide? We wouldn't want to argue that such knowledge is irrelevant, but it doesn't seem right to say that it's the only basis, either. Suppose, for the sake of argument, that you just found out you have Alzheimer's disease and your doctor has advised you to appoint a proxy for health care, as nothing can be done to prevent your becoming severely demented. Suppose too that you have a loving spouse and three adult children, who live nearby and with whom you have a very close relationship. Now suppose that a total stranger approached you and told you, perfectly truthfully, that she had the ability to know with one hundred percent accuracy what you will want when you are in the late stages of dementia. Would you appoint her as your proxy, in preference to your spouse or children?

Some people, of course, might leap at the opportunity. But many would hesitate for a good while before accepting, and some would reject it altogether. If the authority of proxy decisionmakers really is merely a matter of what they know, then hesitation in the face of this offer, seems curious, perhaps irrational. But there is a reason why the idea of the stranger, no matter how knowledgeable and benevolent, makes some of us uneasy; it has something to do with the nature of the right to refuse medical treatment for *oneself.*

Our right to refuse or consent is grounded in the idea that our freedom of agency ought to be respected to the greatest extent compatible with everyone else's exercise of this freedom. Now, it's true that part of the good of free agency is achieving the desired outcome—say, being allowed to die quietly without having to undergo repeated attempts at resuscitation if one is in the final stages of an illness. That's where the proxy's knowledge of the patient's wishes comes in: the outcome is likelier if the proxy knows the patient didn't want resuscitation. Just as important as outcome, however, is the actual exercise of the agency. That these are two distinct things can be shown by considering a different sort of directive regarding one's future affairs: an ordinary Last Will and Testament.

Howards End

The dying and lonely Mrs. Wilcox in E. M. Forster's novel strikes up a friendship with a young woman named Margaret Schlegel, who is kind and good to her. She becomes so fond of Margaret that she bequeaths her beloved home, Howards End, to her new friend. Mr. Wilcox and his children, hating the idea that the house should pass to an outsider, actually suppress Mrs. Wilcox's written directive. Things do turn out all right, of course. By various twists of fate Margaret becomes the second Mrs. Wilcox and so comes into her inheritance despite the family's machinations. At that point, if the ghost of the first Mrs. Wilcox had risen to reproach Mr. Wilcox for not having honored her wishes, he might have replied, "But what you desired has come to pass, so you have no cause for complaint." But he would be wrong; this reply is patently hollow. The first Mrs. Wilcox didn't just want Margaret to *have* Howards End—she wanted to *give* it to her as her gift, as an expression of her agency. The outcome was as she would have wanted it, but it wasn't through her action that the outcome was achieved. Mr. Wilcox failed her not only because he didn't do what she wanted but also because he didn't act as her agent.[19]

Similarly, then, with the proxy for health care. Standing surrogate for another isn't merely a question of doing what someone wants, but of honoring that person's agency in one's own action. To go back to the parents who wonder if they should find other caregivers, wiser and richer than they, to give their child the best possible upbringing, the point is not that our children get the best possible upbringing, but that they get the good of being brought up *by us.* The beloved gets, not the best possible life-partner, but the good of being *this lover's* life-partner. So too at the sickbed. Whether a brother, lover, daughter-in-law will correctly decide what's best for me is not all that's at stake; what's more important is that the decision be made by *this person*—who has lived within the web of relationships that shaped us both, who has been marked by many of the same projects and affections, catastrophes and perspectives. This person, separate from me, nonetheless shares something essential with me and so can stand as an extension of my self. The authority to exercise agency for me, then, comes from this proximity—not merely from special knowledge, not from the community. It is reasoning along these lines that prompts the gerontologist and ethicist Joanne Lynn to explain "Why I Don't Have a Living Will"—why the outcome of the treatment decision matters less to her than who decides. [20] At this point, we can invoke our first use of the stars we're steering by: *Family members aren't replaceable by similarly (or better) qualified people.*

DAD DESIGNATES A PROXY

Seth Kaufman checked in to a large, downtown Chicago hospital for a complete GI series. Certain foods had been disagreeing violently with him lately, and his doctor wanted to rule out as many possibilities as she could before settling on a diagnosis of irritable bowel syndrome. On admission he was given a packet of material to read, including information about the Patient Self-Determination Act—a federal law requiring institutions to explain to patients the laws in their state about treatment directives, should the patient become incompetent. The brochure informed him that he had the right to choose someone to make medical decisions for him, in case he ever lost the capacity to do it for himself. He thought about that, and after talking things over with the health care planning nurse and, next day, with his doctor, he filled out a health care proxy form.

That afternoon his son Mike, a physician at the same hospital, came by to see him. As he approached the door to his father's room, Mike saw his mother, in tears, walking hurriedly down the corridor. He ran to catch up with her.

"What's wrong, Ma? Dad's going to be just fine, you know."

His mother shook her head. "It isn't that. It's just—oh, I'm being silly, that's all. It's his decision and I know it, but it still makes me feel bad."

"What decision? What's he done?"

"He appointed your cousin Ruthie to be his proxy if he ever needs one."

"Ruthie? Why Ruthie? Nobody in the family can stand her."

"I know, but they told your dad he should pick the person who was best qualified, and he didn't want to pick you because you might have to disagree with his doctors and you need to stay on good terms with them. Ruthie's a lawyer, so he thought she'd be second best."

Mike put his arm around her shoulder. "And you wish he'd picked you."

His mother couldn't speak through the tears she was attempting to contain, but she nodded her head.

"Well, the whole thing's ridiculous. You two have been happily married for thirty-five years, and you've always done everything together. Of course you should be the one to make decisions for him. You know how Dad is—he was probably just trying to fill out the form the way he thought he was supposed to. How about if I go talk to him?"

By focusing exclusively on the question of expertise, Mr. Kaufman had neglected the importance of intimacy in medical decisionmaking, and so sent his wife a message he presumably didn't mean to send. Not that respect for intimacy calls for indifference to Mr. Kaufman's wishes. We will suppose that the Kaufmans, along with his physician, discussed in general terms the conditions under which Mr. Kaufman would want to refuse treatment. Would he want ventilator support if he were in the final stages of a fatal disease? Would he want artificial nutrition and hydration if he were in a persistent vegetative state? What about antibiotics if he were demented but in no danger of dying? A real advantage to formally appointing a proxy is that it offers an opportunity to think through one's wishes, aloud, in the presence of the people most concerned to hear them. But if Mike Kaufman was able to persuade his father to appoint Mrs. Kaufman rather than Cousin Ruthie, it would probably be because he managed to call his father out of the unfamiliar, expertise-driven world of medicine and reinsert him into a more familiar context.

Carefully talking things over, of course, is precisely what can't be done in the case of patients who were never competent. For these patients, if we are right about the significance of the family's ability to mark its own in fundamental ways, the fact that **Family members aren't replaceable by similarly (or better) qualified people** takes on a special meaning.

THE SELFLESS

Everybody in their Brooklyn neighborhood called him Hammer. He was Mrs. Henry Green's no-good son, who couldn't hold a steady job and hung out with his friends on the street. He said he was getting some musicians together for a steel-drum band, but his mother couldn't see that much had come of it beyond the drum, which he played at home and sometimes, when she wouldn't give him any money, took down into the subways and played there for loose change. In his twenty-two years of living Hammer, had picked up street education, an HIV infection, and a nice young woman who bore him a son, Arjuna, and shortly thereafter died of AIDS.

Arjuna was now three years old and he too was dying. He had been in and out of the hospital many times in the last year for treatment of various opportunistic infections and twice for pneumocystis pneumonia. His grandmother was good to him and took care of him, and for all her complaints against Hammer, she could see that his little boy had enough of a hold on him to keep him from drifting away altogether. When Arjuna was between hospital visits, Hammer hung around home a little more, and played his drum to the boy. He used to show Arjuna how to make tunes by hitting the different areas on the drum's surface, but now Arjuna was mostly too listless to want to play himself. He liked to listen, though, and lately Mrs. Green had taken to permitting Hammer's no-good friends to bring two other drums into the apartment for rehearsal sessions, since Arjuna seemed to do better then.

Arjuna was back in the hospital again, this time for a fungus infection that had gotten into his bronchial tubes and lungs. The intravenous medicine gave him fever and chills and he cried whenever the nurse came to administer it, or when the lab technician came around to draw more blood. Hammer, who hated hospitals, wouldn't come to visit him, and while this was a constant source of friction between him and Mrs. Green, the pediatrician couldn't help suspect that Hammer was trying not to think about his own bondage to the disease that would almost surely kill him after it finished killing his son.

When Arjuna was stable enough to go home, the pediatrician warned that it might be only a matter of days before the boy would have to come back. Although there was always hope that they could keep him going for a while yet, he said, Arjuna was likely to die soon. "Then I won't bring him back," said Mrs. Green. "Every time I do, you've got to hurt him—don't seem like there's any way you can help it. Let me keep him at home and take care of him like you taught me. He's got his daddy there, and maybe he likes to hear the music. Maybe he'd have played the drum like his daddy if he'd had the chance to grow up."

They talked it over. The pediatrician pointed out that aggressive treatment could be stopped without stopping palliative care. He suggested that next time, rather than calling the ambulance, she bring the boy to the emergency room herself and tell the staff that she wanted them to do nothing more than make him comfortable. But he could see she thought

Arjuna was better off at home where he could get the good of his daddy, and he hoped she was right.

He never saw Mrs. Green or her grandson again. But he heard from the social worker that the little boy had died one evening not three weeks later, while Hammer and his friends rehearsed in the front room.

A child as young as Arjuna has only begun the long process of self-formation. One doesn't know what might have become of him had he had the opportunity to grow into adulthood—to be a person of settled preferences and values, with his own particular outlook on life. Yet what he might have become isn't totally opaque, either. Because families leave their mark on the individuals within them, there is a window into the natures of those whose selves are incomplete. The window into Arjuna's self is a tiny one, smudged and dim, but his grandmother looked into it when she spoke of Arjuna's growing up to be a drummer like his father. With little else to guide her, she made use of the family's ability to imprint itself on its children as she tried to decide what medical treatment would be best for him.

The active principle in the law and in medicine for people who are too ill to make their own treatment decisions has been, "When in doubt, treat." Physicians, driven by the technological imperative (that is, the view that we have the technology, so we should use it), by their reluctance to give in to disease and death, and by the fear of lawsuits, have practiced with a bias toward overtreatment. A proper understanding of the family's role in decisionmaking can help caregivers share their power and (not incidentally) provide a climate within the health care system that is more conducive to good medical practice. What sometimes happens instead is that medical facilities and the courts join forces to override the family's wishes even when there is no question that those wishes conform with what a now-incompetent patient repeatedly stated she would have wanted.

In September of 1992, for example, a middle-level court in the state of New York ruled that a family would have to pay over $100,000 to a nursing home that refused to permit the removal of a feeding tube in a woman who was in a persistent vegetative state, even though the woman, Mrs. Elbaum, had many times extracted promises from her family that she wouldn't be kept alive in such a condition, and her husband had repeatedly directed that the tube be removed. The court found that, because there was no living will or formally appointed proxy, it was up to the court—not the nursing home—to decide whether Mrs. Elbaum's prior statements constituted "clear and convincing evidence" of her wishes, that the family had no say in the matter, and that Mr. Elbaum was liable for medical expenses incurred while the case went to court.[21]

This is an unfortunate decision in a number of respects, not least in that it reinforces the notion that the basic drive of medicine should be to keep people alive no matter what. But even worse is the assumption that close family are irrelevant—at least, when they don't pose an active threat—in determining the fate of an incompetent patient.

Not that familial decisions for those who lack capacity will always proceed smoothly. A major hitch occurs when a patient's relatives are remote, disengaged, or nonexistent. What if, for example, the patient has only two family members—a sister who suffers from schizophrenia and an aunt whom he hasn't seen in twenty years? In cases of this kind the health care team is likely to look to kith rather than kin, seeking a neighbor, friend, business colleague, or other such person who knows the patient and cares about him. Everyone has his daily haunts; when a person seems to have neither friend nor relation it might be possible to locate a cafe where he took most of his meals. Bartenders are a not uncommon source of information about patients who have no other ties.

When family members disagree about what's best to be done, the catastrophe of illness or injury is only compounded. Whatever rifts already exist within the family can easily be exacerbated; catastrophic illness in children, for example, can break a troubled marriage, and the family then typically reconfigures with an absent father and a mother who remains to give the needed care.[22] At times like this it may be especially important to try to protect the family's crumbling integrity, but not if the patient must be scapegoated to do it. An overly romantic view of the family might lead to the temptation to compromise the patient's interests, while an overly cynical view might declare irrelevant anything *but* the patient's interests. But even where there is agreement that her interests ought to be the guiding factor in making treatment decisions, there is likely to be disagreement about just what those interests are.

Consider this story:

PARENTS OR PARTNER: WHO CARES?

Sharon Kowalski was twenty-three when she and Karen Thompson exchanged rings and promised to love each other the rest of their lives. Four years later, in 1983, a car accident left Sharon brain-damaged and quadriplegic, stripped of her short-term memory. She still remembered Karen, however, and the fact that she was a lesbian.

She never told her parents this, perhaps because she feared their reaction. When Karen, who is a professor of physical education at St. Cloud State University in Minnesota, tried to visit Sharon in her nursing home, Mr. and Mrs. Kowalski forbade the visits and, in 1985, obtained a court order to prohibit them. Relations between the Kowalskis and Karen were hostile from the outset, and did not improve when, in 1984, she tried and failed to get legal guardianship of Sharon.

Her visitation rights were restored in 1988, but in 1990, when Mr. Kowalski's health failed and he could no longer carry out his duties, the court appointed a third party—a friend of the Kowalski family—to be Sharon's guardian. The judge denied guardianship to Karen because the Kowalskis threatened to have nothing more to do with their daughter if her friend Karen were appointed; the court also expressed concern at Karen's acknowledgment that she has had sexual relationships with other women and might continue to do so even if she were appointed.

The case became a *cause célèbre* among gay rights groups and advocates of rights for the disabled, who in 1988 organized demonstrations in twenty-one cities, proclaiming "National Free Sharon Kowalski Day." It was not until December of 1991 that a Minnesota appeals court awarded custody to Karen. The court noted that Sharon's caregivers agreed she consistently indicated she wanted to return to St. Cloud to live with Karen, and that she cried after visits from her partner. It also noted that Karen's house is completely accessible by wheelchair, allowing Karen to provide the necessary care at home. As the director of the American Civil Liberties Union's Lesbian and Gay Rights Project observed when the battle was over, "This case exemplifies the difficulties lesbians and gay men have in safeguarding our relationships. The remarkable thing about this case is not that Karen Thompson finally won guardianship, but that it took her seven years to do so, when guardianship rights for a heterosexual married couple would be taken for granted."[23]

If Sharon had been conventionally married the presumption would have been that her husband's judgment concerning what was best for her carried more weight than her parents', and that he had not only the right but the obligation to look after her carefully and well. That was precisely the presumption missing in this case. Because the bond between the two women wasn't recognized in law, Sharon's parents failed to see its moral force.

But suppose lesbianism were not at issue—suppose the Kowalskis' animus against Sharon's partner were driven, not by homophobia, but by social snobbery or some other prejudice for which they couldn't hope to receive a judge's encouragement. In that case they might be equally unwilling to come to terms with her partner. They might well be tempted to do what the Kowalskis actually did do once the courts stopped providing them legal remedy: sever relations with their daughter altogether. Victorian melodramas to the contrary, though, American society has never countenanced parents' disowning their children. Here we have another star to steer by: *Family members are stuck with each other.*

We will argue for this proposition more carefully when we explore parental and filial duties in the next chapter; for now it may be enough to suggest that the love parents are obligated to provide their young children encumbers all the parties involved in a set of further obligations—fidelity among them. It's wrong to sever the bond merely because Sharon is grown. Especially if she then is needy and vulnerable, her parents are bidden to stay connected to their daughter, and to accommodate themselves as best they can to the important intimate relationships she has formed elsewhere. Even if they suspect her spouse or partner to be of bad character, their own lives and that of their daughter might be better for sustained attempts to create an atmosphere of mutual respect and support.[24]

When the Patient Has Some Voice

The role of parents is perhaps even more troublesome when the child is not as helpless as Sharon Kowalski. The capacity of a normal child to make good medical decisions on her own behalf is not totally absent even at the age of five; by the time the child is seventeen her decisions are usually neither better nor worse than a full-grown adult's. Parental involvement here, as elsewhere in a child's life, must accommodate the child's increasing maturity: parents share their power as their children become old enough to wield it for themselves. Medical decisionmaking for children, then, takes place within the context of the child's upbringing, where it constitutes one strand in the broader patterns of moral formation that are an ongoing process of family life.

To save the life of a family member, it can be perfectly appropriate for parents to permit—or perhaps even insist—that a child undergo non-therapeutic medical interventions, at least if these interventions are no more than slightly less safe than the risks she runs in day-to-day life.[25] She may be expected to contribute bone marrow to a sibling, for example, if she is in the best position to provide it. In this way, parents can teach the child to respond to human need, as well as underscore her importance to the family. But it's essential that she *be* a member of the family unit; such sacrifices may be exacted only if she is a citizen and not a slave of the community she serves. If her immediate family neglects or abuses her, they forfeit any special moral claim on her when they are in need; if there is a genetic tie but no other, as might be the case with tissue donation to a half-sibling whom the child doesn't know the star to steer by—**Intimacy produces special responsibilities**—is not present, and the request to donate becomes inappropriate.

Insofar as a child belongs to himself, he may not be asked to make sacrifices on another's behalf when there is a good chance that doing so will cause him irreparable harm. Nor can he be coerced without adequate explanation, loving support, and enough time (if possible) to adapt himself to the exigencies of the situation. In addition, to the extent possible, the burden must not fall disproportionately upon him, but be shared by others in the family. Even if they cannot donate tissue, other members can express their own solidarity in the form of time spent with the child or special care and attention.

When the question is one of medical treatment that benefits the child herself, the degree of power she should have over the decision to accept or refuse it depends very largely on her own medical sophistication and maturity of judgment. A chronically ill child is more likely to be capable of making a good decision at the age of ten than an ordinarily robust child is at twelve: the ten-year-old who has been on kidney dialysis for four years has both a wider and a more profound experience of illness and bodily awareness than the child who has never been seriously ill. Because good parents share their power, they also share their knowledge with the child. In cooperation with the health care team they must disclose (in language the child can understand) the nature of the illness, how it tends to run its course, and what the outcome is likely to be. It takes courage to tell a five-year-old that she will soon die, but if this is not done the child faces death alone, with the additional burden of cooperating in a conspiracy of silence that requires her to take care of her caregivers' feelings.[26]

DR. HUNTER'S DILEMMA

Dr. Hunter was gray-haired and courtly, a slender little man given to three-piece suits and bow ties, for thirty years a pediatrician in a group practice in Nashville, Tennessee. Janet Green, fourteen years old, was a patient of his. He'd known Janet all her life, having taken care of her and her younger brother ever since they were born. He and his wife and the Greens all attended the same African Methodist Episcopal church. He liked Janet. She was a smart girl, in the honor society at high school, and as best he recalled, she was a pretty mean tennis player. She was getting to be a very attractive young lady.

This particular day Janet's dad brought her into the doctor's office because he thought she might have stomach flu. Dr. Hunter caught a glimpse of him in the waiting room, patiently looking over some business papers, as Janet came into the examining room.

She sat quietly on the table, obediently stripped to the waist and clutching the paper gown to her chest. She wouldn't look at him. He asked her how she was feeling and scanned her chart. Temperature, blood pressure—everything was normal. "But you don't feel good?"

She shook her head, looking straight down at her lap.

"You've been throwing up?"

She nodded.

"How long has that been going on?"

She chewed her lip, as if her grades for the semester depended on the answer. He was about to ask her again when she lifted her head and looked him full in the face. "Promise you won't tell anybody," she whispered.

"Tell anybody what?"

"Just promise."

"Honey, I can't just promise without knowing what I'm promising, but you can trust me. We're old friends, sure enough."

She started to cry.

Dr. Hunter wasn't born yesterday, as he was fond of pointing out. He handed her a tissue and asked, "When was your last period?"

"I don't know—a long time ago. I don't keep track."

"Well, let's do a pregnancy test and see if you've been doing all this worrying for nothing."

The urine sample tested positive for beta-hcg, and a blood test confirmed it. Janet Green was definitely pregnant. About ten weeks along, from what Dr. Hunter could piece together by talking further with her. "Who's the fellow?"

"Akkim Jones—he's a junior. Tomorrow's our six-months' anniversary."

"Did you take any kind of precautions?"

"No. Akkim doesn't like the way condoms feel and it's not as if we did it all that often, anyway."

"You did it often enough," Dr. Hunter observed wryly.

Janet started to cry again. "I don't want my parents to find out. They'd just die. They're so proud of me and they're hoping I can get scholarships to go to college, and having this baby would just mess everything up. Don't tell them. Please don't tell them. Can't you give me an abortion so they won't find out what I did?"

The question of teenage abortion poses yet another set of problems for those in authority over a child. The Office of Technology Assessment, a federal government agency, reports that in 1988 in the United States, fifty-three percent of girls aged fifteen to nineteen had had sexual intercourse; of those, eleven percent of girls in that age group were pregnant the year before. In 1990 it was estimated that four out of ten girls become pregnant before the age of twenty, which works out to a rate of one million pregnancies per year. Of these, about half are brought to term while the other half end in abortion. Unmarried mothers under the age of fifteen number ten thousand per year.[27]

Given a cultural climate that promotes sexual activity as an important part of a young person's social development, a sex-gender system that valorizes sexual prowess in men and sexual attractiveness to men in women, and a society that denies teenagers any serious or responsible role in contributing to the common weal, we can hardly wonder at these statistics. Adolescence is a time when there is a natural interest in expanding one's relationships in the broader community, and in assessing one's family from the perspective of a newly gained maturity. Because these impulses typically combine to set up a distance between a teenager and the rest of her family, a discovery of pregnancy will not necessarily be the sort of thing she is prepared to disclose to her parents (although she might tell a sister.) She will, of course, be even less inclined to reveal her condition if the pregnancy is the result of sexual abuse by her father or brother, or if she has experienced violence at home.

Although under common law a minor can't receive health services without parental consent, certain exceptions have been established by the legislatures, state courts, and the Supreme Court. Exceptions fall into three categories: for emergencies; for emancipated minors; and for reproductive health services, including abortion, contraception, and treatment of sexually transmitted disease. The exceptions vary widely from state to state, and in some states a judge's permission is required in the absence of parental consent. In some states the child doesn't need her parent's consent, but the parents have to be notified.

Whether the child ought to end the pregnancy, carry it to term but give the baby up for adoption, or keep the baby depends on the her age, family situation, economic status, and myriad other particulars too numerous for the broad ship of the law to navigate properly. That being the case, it is all the more important that the child's advisors—particularly her physician, but also other adults who have her interests at heart—help her to understand as fully as possible the ethical issues at stake. It is crucial that Dr. Hunter avoid the pitfall of romanticizing Janet's family: if she believes she must have an abortion without her parents' knowledge, Dr. Hunter should explore with her the reasons, but must respect her ultimate decision, no matter how much her likes her parents or how badly he thinks she's misjudged them.

The reason, as Alison M. Jaggar explains, is that "decisions should be made by those, and only by those, who are importantly affected by them."[28] Given the imbalance of power between the genders, we cannot say with certainty that in any given act of intercourse the woman or girl was not coerced. The bodily consequences of pregnancy, ranging from restrictive to life-threatening, are grave enough that a means of avoiding those consequences must always be available. Moreover, the fact that our sex-gender system imposes by far the greater share of the burden of rearing children on mothers rather than fathers is by itself a compelling reason for ensuring that girls and women have a means of stopping those responsibilities before they start. Janet will not have made her decision to abort in unfettered freedom, any more than she chose in unfettered freedom to engage in sexual intercourse in the first place. However, for the reasons just enumerated and because it is an enormous responsibility to bring another human being into the world, the adults to whom Janet turns must be careful to help her set her decision within the context of her own life plan, not her parents' life plan or anyone else's.

Had the decision gone the other way, Janet's parents would have to have been consulted, to follow Jaggar's principle fully. That is, if Janet, at fourteen, were inclined to undertake this pregnancy and give birth, it would no longer be she alone who was importantly affected by the decision. Her parents would not only become grandparents, but surrogate parents, as Janet would be too young to be entrusted with the baby's care. They may not violate Janet's person by forcing her to have an abortion, but they are certainly permitted to object, cajole, reason with, plead, and use other strong forms of moral suasion to attempt to get her to change her mind.

The Competent Patient's Choices

What we've outlined so far are special considerations having to do with patients who can't make their own choices, or whose ability to do so is limited and whose choices must be assisted by others. Now we move to a discussion of decisionmaking for oneself. When I am in the final stages of breast cancer, should I insist that everything possible be done to fight it? When diabetes produces gangrene in my foot, should I refuse to permit amputation even though I will die without it? Should I hazard the possibility of unknown side-effects and enroll myself in a clinical trial of an experimental drug to control obsessive-compulsive disorder? What about coronary bypass surgery? Do-Not-Resuscitate orders? Long-term care options?

Decisions of this kind have two components: who decides, and what is decided. An ethics of the family challenges the "who" and adds a new dimension to the what.

A third star helps us steer here. The fact that *Families are ongoing stories* means that decisions can be set within the context of the individual's story as well as within the family's broader story. The narrative tradition of a family:

1. identifies everybody who has a stake in a decision;
2. provides a basis for decisionmaking that isn't arbitrary, but rests on ethically salient, although highly particular, considerations.

Let's take these points, which are applicable to any kind of decisionmaking, one at a time.

Thinking of a family as a story helps us to recognize its scope—that is, it helps us to identify all the characters who play a major role in it. Members may not be excluded from consideration just because other family members dislike them, or disagree with them, or refuse to recognize their connection with the patient. If one thinks of the family as a novel in which the patient's story is but one chapter, one can more easily pick out the leading characters. Sharon Kowalski's parents, for example, might more easily have seen that her partner Karen was in point of fact a member of her family—one who had a strong interest in the decisions to be made.

They forgot the patient's point of view, but that is not the only view that is relevant to the family's story. Failing an omniscient narrator, the story must always be told from the point of view of one member of the family or another, but not always from the same one. A switch in perspective must be possible if there is to be any genuine understanding among its members.

But the narrative does more than identify the stakeholders; it also asserts that the *quality* of the decision matters as well as who is making it. I may have a right to privacy, for example, or to discretion over my own body, yet I may exercise these rights in a nasty way—as when I have a vasectomy without talking it over with my wife, even though I know she wants more children. Thinking about her story as a part of my own underscores how rights can conflict with responsibilities to others. Or (in a different kind of problem) I might have three or four options open to me, all of which are permissible and none of which, if exercised, would make me a scoundrel, but I don't know how to pick among them except by flipping a coin. By thinking of my family story, I have a nonarbitrary basis for decisionmaking: I can look to my own and my family's patterns of past choices to provide guidance for a present decision. I needn't follow the pattern, but if I am aware of what it is and it seems good, I can choose to ratify it. I can modify it if necessary, or, if it is a pattern I find morally discreditable, repudiate it altogether. Here's an example of how this works.

BUSINESS AS USUAL

Alvin Murphy is an engineer in a large food-processing plant in Denver. His is technically a white-collar job, but he is never happier than when scrambling up on a girder with a wrench in his pocket, trying to figure out what is causing the number-four engine to quiver, or why a conveyor belt is slipping. He has kept the plant at Universal Foods going for twenty years, and he is now Chief Engineer, with three engineers under him. He's always worked very hard at his job, possibly because he's more comfortable with machines than with people.

Partly because he was so focused on his job, he let his home life slip. His wife grew increasingly discontented with his neglect, and after ten years she ended their marriage. He agreed to let her have custody of their two boys, Pete and Charlie. Charlie, now fifteen, recently announced he needed to live with his dad for a while, and that's been going quite well. Alvin generally doesn't get home until after eight at night, which gives Charlie plenty of elbow room for school and tinkering with his car; Charlie, like his father, enjoys the company of machinery.

Over the last year or so Alvin has had some bad bouts with his back—the most recent one being so painful that he was laid up in bed for a week. His doctor has told him he must lose weight, and that he can't be swinging around on the girders anymore—it's time to leave that sort of work to the younger men. But Alvin has been trying to get along on muscle relaxants and pain killers, refusing to acknowledge that he must make changes in the way he lives.

The treatment decision facing Alvin presents an opportunity for him to practice what Margaret Walker calls strong moral self-definition.[29] That is, Alvin can use the particulars of his own life story to construct a moral persona for himself. This process of moral self-definition takes place in three steps:

1. Alvin weighs the particulars of his situation in terms of his more general values: what do his passion for his job, his failed marriage, his pleasant but distant relationship with his son mean in the light of his broader beliefs and principles? How are these particulars relevant to the decision about treatment for his bad back?

2. Alvin discerns a course of action expressing a certain strength and type of commitment to these particulars. He can sustain the old course of his life, letting things drift along with Charlie and coping as best he can with his ailing body, but putting highest value on his work, or he can chart a new course, reconfiguring his job to eliminate some of the stress on his back and assigning a higher weight to his relationship with his son. He chooses, we will suppose, to accept a new job description. In doing this he is saying something to himself about his commitment to the job as well as about how much he values his relationship to his son. This kind of discernment is what it means to define oneself morally.

3. Alvin at the same time is endorsing for the future the connection between the particulars of his life and the judgment by which he assigns these particulars their relative value. He is beginning a moral track-record for himself, declaring by his actions that he wishes to alter the previous course of his life and (what is just as important) that he is setting a new course for himself. In this step, because he is committing himself to certain values for the future, he is setting up legitimate expectations on the part of others that he will follow the plot outline he has established: Charlie would justifiably be disappointed if, having scaled back his job, Alvin now spends even less time with the boy than he did before.

Sometimes the alternatives are not all acceptable, even when we can come up with persuasive justifications for them.

IT'S MY HEART ATTACK

Molly Cobb, fifty-seven years old, is an executive secretary in a small city in Virginia. Having married late, she was widowed when her only child, Susan, was a toddler. She has a number of brothers and sisters living nearby with their own families, as well as a network of aunts and uncles and cousins. Molly is quite attached to her family, but also somewhat exasperated by their well-meaning and officious attempts to meddle in her affairs. She is a rather private person, brought up in the Southern female tradition of making light of one's own troubles and directing one's energy and attention toward the welfare of others.

Her daughter Susan is now a freshman in high school—a happy, intelligent, and well-liked student, vice-president of her class and active in a number of extracurricular activities. Susan and Molly enjoy a good relationship, in part, Molly thinks, because she made a rule when Susan's father died that she would never burden Susan with her own cares or responsibilities; she would take care of Susan, and not the other way around.

Last summer when Susan was at camp in North Carolina, Molly suffered a mild heart attack. She felt fine afterward, but her doctor put her on a regimen of diet, moderate exercise, and prescribed medications. She insisted that her doctor, who is also her friend, keep the episode confidential, explaining that her family would make nuisances of themselves if they knew about it. "And besides, I don't want to scare Susan."

During the past six months she has stuck to her medical regimen faithfully, but she is sometimes troubled by angina and shortness of breath. At a checkup her doctor urges her to let Susan know about her heart disease, pointing out that if she suffered another attack and Susan were prepared to expect it, she would be far less traumatized than if she were kept in ignorance.

"No," Molly insists. "It's *my* heart attack. What's the good of talking about a patient's right to privacy if the patient can't exercise it as she sees fit?"

"But Molly, think of Susan!"

"I am thinking of Susan. Do I have a right to privacy or don't I?"

"You do, but—"

"Then I'm not doing anything wrong."

Is Molly doing something wrong? We think so. In the first place, we're not altogether certain that rights-talk is appropriate to intimate relationships, and not because people within them don't have rights. Rights can be assigned, but once you have done it it's not clear you've done anything much. That is, Molly might have a general right to privacy—of the sort that keeps her grocer or the government from intruding into her personal affairs—but Susan is a part of her personal affairs, and sorting out to what degree she may be privy to her mother's secrets calls for a fine-grained judgment that must be guided by something much subtler than the idea of rights. Molly has a right to privacy; Susan, as probable emergency caretaker, has a right to know her mother's health status. The rights are in conflict, and what then?

What's missing from this way of approaching the issue is any acknowledgment of the special claims people have on each other within a setting of intimacy. Intimacy exists in a sphere of such densely clustered particulars that the relations among the people involved can't easily be captured by talk of rights. Intimates belong to each other as well as to themselves, and this belonging has moral consequences. When a person shuts another out of an important process or event, she is saying something about what she takes the degree of intimacy between them to be. Here again the idea of family as narrative is helpful: it behooves Molly to think of her life with Susan as a story, asking herself whether the course of the narrative to date is such that this insistence on privacy is warranted, or whether, on the contrary, Susan may legitimately expect more openness and trust from her mother. Is it time to modify the course of self-effacement Molly has always pursued? What particulars of her life does she now devalue if she ratifies the old course? And in what ways has *Susan* defined herself morally so as to warrant Molly's confidences?

In the story of Alvin and Charlie we offered a method of making nonarbitrary decisions when faced with a number of valid alternatives. In the story of Molly and Susan we explored the idea that people in an intimate relationship have special moral claims on each other—claims that cut into one's personal rights. In the next story we want to see if we can set a limit on those special claims.

THE NASTY OLD MAN

Isaiah and Davida Grigg were married in southern Utah in 1946, just after Isaiah returned from the war in the Pacific. They bought a small ranch and began raising cattle, and soon they were raising children as well. There were six young Griggs in all, and all were brought up in the old fashioned way, to respect and obey their father according to the example their mother set them. Isaiah thought of himself as an Old Testament patriarch, and he ruled with a firm hand.

111

As the years went by the children left home, one by one, glad to throw off the burdensome yoke of their father's domination. For their mother's sake, most of them maintained some sort of tie with the parental home; she had often stood between them and a whipping when they were young, and she had comforted them with cookies and kind words when the whipping came anyway. It was not that Isaiah was a brute, but he was a stern man with rigid ideas of right and wrong, and he would do his duty even if his children failed in theirs.

Davida was a good wife to him, working as hard as he did to make the ranch pay. She was a loving grandmother, a faithful churchgoer, and an excellent housewife. She could always be counted on when a neighbor was sick or in need, and she smoothed things over when Isaiah's increasing harshness affronted the ranch hands or neighbors.

Just before his seventy-second birthday, Isaiah suffered a small stroke, which left him somewhat forgetful and rather more irritable. More of the work of the ranch now fell to Davida, and the children grew concerned as they watched their mother overwork herself to keep everything going to Isaiah's satisfaction.

Isaiah's health grew progressively worse: he became diabetic, his blood pressure was high, and he developed phlebitis in his left leg. None of this improved his temper, which he relieved by haranguing his wife and occasionally striking her. When he began to suffer from urinary incontinence the children called a family council.

Judy, the oldest daughter, assumed the role of spokeswoman. "We know you want to keep things as they are, Dad," she said, "but it's time to start thinking about a nursing home. Mom can't go on like this and if she keeps trying she'll make herself ill. Now, we've been looking into it and there's a very nice place in St. George, which is a retirement town anyway and there are lots of people your age—"

But her father would not let her finish. "I won't have it. My place is here and your mother's place is beside me. She'll do her duty by me as she always has done and that's the end of it."

"But I can't," Davida told him. "The children are right—your care is getting to be too much for me. If it's the money you're worrying about you needn't be, because we have enough invested and we'll have to sell the ranch one of these days anyway. Or if you like there's the VA hospital. We just thought St. George would suit you better."

"You'll do as I say. I won't be turned out of my own home and I'll be damned if anybody else looks after me. That's your job."[30]

What do we make of this? In the first place, here we see a clear-cut difference between the ethics of medicine and the ethics of the family: providing health care is a primary end of medicine, but it is a secondary end for families. Davida's primary role as wife is not to provide health care to her husband, but to build a life together with him. This difference between the two systems means that Isaiah may legitimately demand care from a private nursing home (so long as he can pay for it) or from a VA facility, but he may not impose this duty on family members. As a matter of fact, patient preference doesn't override all other considerations even in a professional setting: health care providers have never been obliged to give treatment that is inappropriate according to the standards of their profession. In families, even where the treatment is appropriate, the question of who is to provide needed care can't be dictated unilaterally.

Secondly, Isaiah fails to acknowledge that a family structure in which unpaid care is demanded of women solely because they are women is unfair. It imposes an unpleasant and demanding job on wives for no better reason than that women have traditionally been forced to do it, but to perpetuate this pattern is to assume that women should be coerced, without compensation, into doing work no one else wants to do, just because they are women. That is an outrageous assumption.

Thirdly, if we use the family's narrative to guide our analysis, we will note that Davida has generally placed Isaiah's interests ahead of her own, at no small cost to herself. Simple justice suggests that it's her turn to be considered first. If we look at it in this light, she should be excused from caring for Isaiah strictly on his own terms and ought to have lavish amounts of familial care herself when the time comes.

If Molly doesn't have an unfettered right to privacy, and Isaiah doesn't have an unfettered right to the treatment of his choice, either from his family or from health care professionals, what about other rights? It's widely believed that people do have an absolute right, rooted in the fundamental principle of informed consent, to *refuse* treatment. But if you take families seriously this right too must sometimes yield to responsibilities toward others—especially where the stakes for the patient are relatively low and the cost of the alternative to invasive treatment is very high.

In fact, even when the stakes for the patient are high, there are occasional cases where it might be wrong to refuse treatment. In *In re President & Directors of Georgetown College, Inc.*, the court compelled a Jehovah's Witness to receive a blood transfusion against her wishes, arguing that the state had a compelling interest in protecting her seven-month-old child's right to continued maternal care.[31] We don't endorse the court's decision. In a society where women are devalued, silenced, and too often pressed into unrelieved caregiving because men will not do it, no court should force a woman to receive even life-sustaining treatment against her will for the sake of her child. But that doesn't mean the woman was right. Her responsibility to the child, which derives in part from having brought it into existence, might well (especially if the father is dead or unable to care for the baby) take precedence over even a strongly held religious principle.

Where the stakes are higher for family members than for the patient, we can see more clearly the trouble with exercising one's right to refuse treatment. If, for example, a kidney stone can be removed by catheterization for a fraction of what it costs to have it pulverized by lithotripsy, and if the family is uninsured for lithotripsy, the patient may justly be censured for insisting that the family's savings be wiped out simply so that he may refuse catheterization. In fact, John Hardwig would go a step further: "In many cases family members have a greater interest than the patient in which treatment option is exercised. In such cases, the interests of family members often ought to *override* those of the patient." Why? Because "to be close is to no longer have a life entirely your own to live entirely as you choose. To be part of a family is to be morally required to make decisions on the basis of thinking about what is best for all concerned, not simply what is best for yourself." Simple fairness, Hardwig believes, dictates that all those with an interest in the decision be taken into account as it is made.[32]

This is an upsetting and radical claim for the profession. It means, first of all, that families should be involved in the decisionmaking process not just as sounding-boards and not just as a source of patient-centered love and support, but in their own right. Rather than being instructed by the health care team to focus on what is best for the patient, family members should be encouraged to get their own interests, fears, and preferences on the table. They should be treated not just as means to the patient's ends, but as ends in themselves.

But that is not all. If we have the courage to follow the argument from fairness to wherever it leads us, we must acknowledge that when a fundamental disagreement arises between the patient and the rest of the family, and no amount of discussion or mediation can resolve it, the health care team might be obliged to try do what the family wants *even though the patient dissents*. If this outcome is *never* permitted, then we are only paying lip service to the idea that families matter.

Now, one objection to this argument might be that we've gotten the premises wrong. It's not true, the objection would go, that all the stakeholders in decisions at the bedside are on the same footing. The suffering, vulnerable patient will always have immeasurably more at stake than anyone else, which is why society thrusts her into a special role and surrounds her with a highly ritualistic panoply of practices, some of which have very little indeed to do with achieving health, but everything to do with protecting the patient from harm. The family must, on this objection, understand and participate in these social rituals of protection or the patient will suffer even further.

A practical, but incomplete, response to this objection would be to note that if all the familial motives and concerns are allowed out into the open, the health care team can see them and assess them for what they are. If instead, as is currently the case, these concerns are driven underground, they are apt to come out subtly, in the form of covert pressure that won't be acknowledged by anyone and so poses a greater threat to the patient.[33]

That response (although we think it is true), isn't fully adequate because it assumes that a patient-centered focus, and not the family's more communal standpoint, is the only safeguard against familial abuse of the vulnerable. It assumes, to put it bluntly, that what the patient rightly fears most is that her family will do her harm as she lies defenseless and ill.

This is an odd assumption. Most families don't use the health care delivery system as a means of mistreating the helpless. Why, then, construct a policy that treats all families as if they did? It might be thought that a default assumption of mistrust is safer, because it does prevent actual abuse and hurts no one where families are loving rather than abusive. But in point of fact, it *does* hurt people in loving families: it courts a real danger of breaking down the intricate network of relationships—already strained by serious illness—within which the patient is situated. Routinely and systematically treating people as if they were adversaries is likely to make them so. At the very least, the default assumption of mistrust sets up emotional barriers among family members at the precise moment when they need all the comfort intimacy can give them.

An analogy: suppose a community became so fearful of sexual molestation that it framed a policy forbidding adults to touch any child without first getting the child's consent. Such a policy would certainly teach children that nonconsensual touching is wrong, which in turn might even diminish the incidence of sexual molestation. But it would also mean that no child would ever receive a spontaneous cuddle or a casual smooch, and as these are an important way for parents to show affection, the constraint would take its toll on the relationship between parent and child. It might even teach children to regard all grownups as potential molesters.

It would seem that the cure is worse than the disease—as it also is, we submit, in the intensive care unit or the nursing home. All the same, physicians and other care providers have a responsibility to shield their patients from abuse. The ethics of their profession doesn't allow them to stand by while a patient is mistreated, much less to collaborate in the mistreatment. How, then, can caregivers avoid such collaboration while at the same time honoring families' claims to respectful and fair consideration?

It would help if caregivers could ask themselves what kind of family they are dealing with—a *Gesellschaft* or a *Gemeinschaft*. The *Gesellschaft* is the corporate model, consisting of an aggregate of persons who come together because that is the best way to maximize their own individual interests. In a *Gemeinschaft*, on the other hand, the purpose is either to achieve some common goal or to experience group solidarity, and individuals act to strengthen that solidarity even if they must compromise their own interests to do so.

A way for health care providers to tell what kind of family they are dealing with is to listen to the decisionmaking process. If the patient or another family member needs to insist on his rights because others are tyrannizing him, the family is a *Gesellschaft*, and the physician's duty is to see if she can't nudge it back in a *Gemeinschaft* direction. If this proves impossible, the dispute must be mediated to take account of the interested parties' individual concerns—or, failing that, adjudicated in court. If, however, the family is loving and solid enough not to need the language of rights, its ability to arrive at consensus should be respected and encouraged.

Suppose, for instance, an eighty-five-year-old patient tells her physician she would rather not have cataract surgery because she's afraid of it, but her adult daughter, with whom she lives, is insistent. She argues that improved sight will not only make her mother happier but will also make life easier for the rest of the family, who have been pressed into service to read to the old lady and help her get around the house. Using the strategy we've just suggested, the physician would resist the impulse to play patient advocate against the daughter and would instead, after being satisfied that the patient was situated within a *Gemeinschaft*, try to do everything she could to persuade the patient to go ahead with the surgery. We aren't arguing that the old lady should be dragged struggling into the operating room, nor are we advocating that the physician play moral cop, taking it upon herself to enforce the maxim that the family's interests should sometimes override the patient's. Rather, we're arguing for a reorientation in the thinking of all the parties involved. Caregivers ought not too quickly to cry abuse; families ought to trust their own judgments as they care for their own; patients ought to remember that **Intimacy produces responsibilities,** and that these may require submitting to beneficial surgery.

If health care professionals continue to view the dominant, patient-centered, interest-maximizing model as the only correct method of making treatment decisions, they may inadvertently turn a *Gemeinschaft* into a *Gesellschaft*, just at the moment when the patient needs most to be in solidarity with those closest to her. Physicians must be careful not to do the family harm; there are better ways to keep patients from familial abuse.

Our suggested reorientation also presupposes, of course, that health professionals will be careful to avoid a circular definition of abuse: if abuse is defined as anything that doesn't maximize the patient's interest, then we are back to an overly cynical view of families and no way of distinguishing between those that pose a risk to patients and those that don't.

Finally, it's important that physicians not measure the impact of this reorientation solely in terms of the medical outcome for the patient. The good of personal self-determination is often more valuable than mere physical health. When caregivers honor the patient's web of intimacy, they may well get a better health outcome, but even when they don't, they have done the right thing. Treatment outcomes, after all, aren't the only, or even the most important, value in life.

If health professionals need to be less cynical about families, it's also important that families resist romanticizing medicine. Families must understand that their expectations of what the doctor can do for the patient will sometimes be unrealistic, either because the family knows little about medicine or because feelings of guilt or desperation are distorting what it does know. Family members must be willing to try to understand the physician's explanations and to ask questions when they aren't sure about what they're being told. They would also, under our reorientation, have an obligation to make their part in the decisionmaking process as "transparent" as possible, voicing their concerns and fears carefully, so that the physician can help them sort out which are realistic and which are not.

"Transparency" is a duty of the physician, too. The notion, which is Howard Brody's, is that the physician will engage in the typical patient-management thought process, only she will do it out loud, in language the patient and her family can understand. [34] This process gives them a better feel for what is certain and for what must be guessed at, what can be hoped for and what cannot, and so lays out the medical constraints within which the treatment goals must be set. If the physician and the rest of the health care team are willing to engage in this kind of openness, and if they encourage patients and families to do the same, the quality of the decision will be much improved.

Decisions about treatment are often difficult, made as they are under conditions of uncertainty. Not all the relevant information can be known; fear, suffering, and guilt compound perplexity. Because these conditions prevail, it's important to keep moral space open in health care institutions—to provide an atmosphere of encouragement and support that permits all parties to the decision to come together to talk things over. [35] In such a setting it is possible to point out salient considerations, to make conceptual distinctions, and to frame decisions so that all the moral principles and values that must be set in the balance become visible. Within this moral space decisionmaking becomes a messy thing. It ought to be. Our vital relationships are messy too.

Chapter Five

When I'm Sixty-Four

THE MEDICINE OF OUR DAY HAS GIVEN US POWERS THAT PEOPLE HAVE longed for, time out of mind: added control over the length of our lives and over the tie between sexuality and reproduction. But the impact of these new powers underscores a warning that is probably as ancient as our longings: be careful what you wish for. You might get it.

As medicine extends the human lifespan in postindustrial societies, those who used to die now grow old—but they are often infirm. At the same time, the size of the family (in part due to medicalized control over conception), has dwindled over the last three decades. The result has been an inverted demographic pyramid, with an increasing number of elderly people supported and cared for by a decreasing number of young adults. This problem, already quite large, is potentially immense. None of the trends that are building this inverted pyramid so threatening to family and community life look to be reversing themselves: more and more people will need health care and other forms of more and more costly social support, and there will be fewer and fewer people to provide the care and bear the costs. Care for the aged has become a matter of serious concern, both as a question of public policy and as a familial dilemma.

Some numbers: the twentieth century has seen an eightfold increase in the number of people over sixty-five years of age; representing only four percent of the population in 1900, they now make up 12.4 percent of all U.S. citizens. The fastest growing age group in the country consists of those over eighty-five, who are twenty-one times as numerous as they were at the turn of the century. In 1965 those over sixty-five outnumbered those under eighteen for the first time in American history—a phenomenon attributable in part to a decline in the birth rate. In the fifty years between 1931 and 1981, the number of women who had borne four or more children dropped from 47.1 percent to 25.5 percent, while in 1979 it was expected that on average a woman would have two children in her lifetime, down from three in 1967. So those who are now over eighty have many fewer children to support them in their old age than their own parents had when they were old. All this adds up to a new challenge for families: adult children now provide a greater amount of care and more difficult care to their parents and parents-in-law for far longer than ever before in history.[1]

Medicine may not be solely responsible for getting families into this fix, but it is without question deeply implicated: it has had a direct and profound impact on the shape of the family. For one thing, the birth-control pill, introduced in the United States in 1960, not only decreased the birth rate but established social expectations that family size was to be a matter of choice. By the same token, medical interventions increased the human lifespan. Antibiotics and improved public health measures lessened the threat of infectious disease; the hygienic reform of American hospitals and better prenatal care greatly reduced the danger of dying in childbirth; improvements in anaesthesia and surgical techniques and the large-scale development of corporate pharmacology have greatly contributed to the lengths of our lives.

In addition to medicine's heavy contribution to the double phenomena of an extended lifespan and a dwindling youthful population, medicine offers its own answers to the condition of old age. As we look to medicine not only to soften the effects of aging but also to conquer it, we have come to see old age as a disease requiring a medical solution.[2] This has yielded some painfully ironic consequences. The medicalization of old age means that we no longer die as often of acute illness—which is to say quickly. Rather we linger, dying of the chronic illnesses which our health care system neither understands well nor can treat with much success, and whose burdens, consequently, fall more heavily on both the old and their families. Caring for the aged tends to be, then, more a familial than a medical concern. Families are still playing one of their standard roles in medically directed dramas: to pick up the pieces left by medical intervention, to provide the caring that medicine can't. But while families are used to this role, the demographic shift they are undergoing threatens to deplete the family's capital of caring.

To explain what we mean by this, we first must dispel some rather stubborn myths. It is not true, for example, that most elderly people end up in nursing homes, unloved and abandoned. Only five percent of those over sixty-five require nursing home care in a given year, and in general this option is the last resort, resisted by families until all other possible alternatives have been exhausted.[3]

It's also untrue that many elderly are all alone in the world. Over four-fifths have at least one adult child, and virtually nobody is totally without kin. Of the ninety-five percent of the elderly who are not in institutions, most live independently, but within an hour's distance of a child. They and their children prefer this "intimacy at a distance" and stay in close touch, calling and visiting at least once a week. [4]

Another myth has it that old people are frequently victimized by their offspring, who, when they aren't plotting to get hold of their money, are mistreating, belittling, and physically neglecting them. Not so. In 1981 the U.S. Select Committee on Aging estimated that four percent of the elderly are victims of abuse in one form or another, but a large and careful study of a random sampling of old people in 1988 indicates that less than one percent are neglected, psychologically abused, or physically mistreated by their children.[5]

A fourth myth tells us that in contemporary America the old are disregarded and considered useless, as outmoded in our postmodern, computerized culture as an old Royal typewriter. As a matter of fact, retirement keeps many old people busier than ever. Indeed, intergenerational exchanges of services are the rule rather than the exception. Grandparents provide seventeen percent of the day-care required for children of working parents, and they also step in to rear their grandchildren (or great-grandchildren) when the parents are absent, dead, or drug-addicted. Furthermore, the elderly give their children and grandchildren money, attention, advice, and services; in times of divorce or illness they provide support and assistance; when families are fragmented they become what is often the only source of unity and stability. As Daniel Callahan observes, "There is evidence to suggest that within the family, the elderly may give more assistance than they receive."[6]

This assistance is of course dependent to some extent on the old person's state of health. Here we should distinguish between the "young-old" (sixty-five to seventy-five), the "old-old" (seventy-five to eighty-five), and the "very old" (over eighty-five). While bodily vigor may well permit even the "very old" to continue to care for others as necessity dictates or desire inclines, it is also true that the elderly are particularly vulnerable to wasting diseases over which medical science has no power. Medicine has made great advances in curing the diseases that produce quick deaths, like heart attacks or pneumonia, but this means that there are now so many more of us to die of Parkinson's or Alzheimer's disease. And these are, of course, precisely the illnesses that require years of familial care.

Who Cares?

But talking of "familial care" obscures some important realities. Who is actually doing the caring? Overwhelmingly it is middle-aged daughters—or daughters-in-law. These are the women Elaine M. Brody calls "women in the middle," who find themselves rearing children and often working for income while they provide care for their own or their husband's aging relatives. Brody's data indicate that while women want the men in the family to assume equal responsibility for care, men don't do it, although they're willing to provide financial help. The belief that caregiving is women's work is so deeply engrained in our culture that it often doesn't occur to women that their husbands or brothers could have taken primary responsibility for their parents' care. Brody reports that even women who don't accept traditional views of women's roles often behave as if they did when it comes to frail elderly relatives. A daughter says: "My two brothers and I are all busy lawyers. But when my mother got sick—she lives in another state—my brothers just assumed that I would be the one to fly out to her. And you know something? I did it." Similarly, when a parent-in-law has no daughter, the obligation for care falls on the daughter-in-law rather than the son. "My husband is an only child," said one, "so there was no one else." Said another with apparently unwitting irony, when asked how *she* came to be her mother-in-law's caregiver, "My husband has two brothers, but he was always the one in the family who took the most responsibility."[7]

The toll this caring takes is sometimes considerable. The physical labor of changing the dirty diapers and wet sheets of incontinent parents, the interrupted sleep so that medications can be given two or three times a night or fears can be calmed, the continual worry that a forgetful parent will leave the stove on or fall and break a bone—these, as bad as they are, are not the hardest burden to bear.

> The most severe impact of caring for a dependent adult appears to be that it is totally monopolizing and without respite, twenty-four hours a day, seven days a week, 365 days a year. . . . There is gradually isolation of the whole family, but particularly the main caregiver. They no longer go out, no longer invite people over, no longer accept invitations, because they cannot leave the dependent person alone and are too nervous about their unpredictable behavior to receive people or to have confidence in substitute care.[8]

Under these circumstances, the caregiver experiences extreme mental and physical fatigue. She has difficulty concentrating, cannot sleep, and often gives up salaried work or switches to part-time work, despite the repercussions this has on future earnings and pensions. Life becomes difficult for the rest of the family too. Marital intimacy is circumscribed and strained; if the caregiver is a gay man or lesbian—a "natural" for the role because the person is not married—the caregiver's partner may find he or she must compete for the caregiver's time and energy, and the relationship languishes because it cannot be tended. Children are reluctant to have their friends visit them for fear the grandparent will do or say something embarrassing; family vacations or outings are put on hold indefinitely.

The question of what we owe our elderly parents has in general been posed in gender-neutral language, setting the terms for the discussion in ways that importantly falsify it. The question of filial obligation must be recast in terms that acknowledge women's pivotal place in it. The investments that have formed the capital of care have largely come out of women's labor, although its depletion threatens the interests of everyone in the family.

Chapter Five

HE'S SO EMBARRASSING

Deirdre Flaherty and Libby Kushner are domestic partners living in a small town in Massachusetts where lesbian couples aren't regarded as particularly strange. With them live Deirdre's twelve-year-old son, Andy, her fourteen-year-old daughter, Felicia, and Libby's elderly father, whom the kids call Grandpa. Deirdre was divorced when Andy was a baby, so the children have never known any other life than this one, in which they have two mothers to bring them up and one grandpa to tell them stories.

Lately, however, Grandpa has been getting increasingly forgetful. He turns on the stove to heat soup for his lunch, and then wanders into the living room under the impression he's already eaten. He asks Andy what time it is and then asks again a few minutes later. When Felicia made a cake to take to the cast party on the closing night of the high school play, it disappeared from the kitchen and was found much later that night, half eaten, on the floor of Grandpa's closet.

"Mother!" Felicia exploded to Libby. "You have GOT to do something about Grandpa. It's not just the cake—it's—well, he's so bizarre! I can't even have my friends over any more."

"Has he been rude to them?"

"No, but he's so embarrassing. Nobody wants to talk to him—especially when he asks the same question over and over. It's uncool even being in the same room with him."

"Yeah," Andy chimed in. "Me'n Doug were trying to play video games yesterday and Grandpa was just weird. Doug even asked me what was the matter with him."

"What did you tell him?" Deirdre wanted to know.

"Well, nothing. I mean, I was pretty embarrassed."

That evening after the children were sent upstairs to do their homework and Grandpa was safely installed in front of the TV, Deirdre and Libby talked it over in the kitchen. The St. Francis home could take him, Libby reported; she had made inquiries. He'd have to face the upheaval sooner or later anyway, but he'd be well looked after there, and it was so important for the children to be able to have a normal social life. They were both at the age where their friendships really mattered.

Deirdre removed her soapy hands from the dishwater and dried them thoughtfully on the towel. "You've said that before and I guess I went along with it, but do you know, I think we've been making a really big mistake. Why aren't we teaching the children to have a little more compassion? Why didn't we tell Andy that he should explain to Doug what it's like to be old and forgetful? Why *can't* Felicia have her friends over? It's not like Grandpa's abusive or nasty—he's perfectly gentle. We don't owe the kids a perfectly smooth social life. I don't think we ought to turn Grandpa out of his home just because the children have to deal with a little embarrassment."

Libby Kushner and Deirdre Flaherty are trying to set the care of an aged parent into the overall context of family life. But in Libby's determination to make life run pleasantly for her children, she is in danger of losing sight of her responsibilities to her father. Deirdre is right to point out that this is his home too; she is also right to remember that *Virtues are learned at our mother's (and father's) knees,* and that she and Libby ought to be in the business of teaching their children compassion. For the children, too, have familial responsibilities, and it's not too soon for them to respond lovingly to their grandfather's need for patience.

Where does the obligation to look after a frail parent or grandparent come from, and how strong an obligation is it? Why shouldn't Libby put her children's interest in having a socially normal household ahead of her father's interest in remaining at home? We'd like to offer Deirdre and Libby some things to think about as they try to sort out what's best for everyone—to provide them with some moral resources for finding their way through this thicket of dilemmas.

While such resources can, in the nature of things, only be general guides, they are nonetheless widely useful. A key resources is an understanding of why generations within a family have obligations to each other at all, and, in particular, what it is that younger generations owe to the old. Understanding where these obligations come from can help us to figure out how much pull they ought to exert on us, relative to our other obligations and aims in life.

What We Owe Our Parents, and Why

Explanations of why we do—or don't—owe our parents anything, and of what the contents of the obligation—if any—might be, can be divided into four groups. The first group consists of theories that base duty on debt:

our parents gave us life and took care of us when we needed care; in return, we owe them care when they are in need. Aristotle and Aquinas both argued this way.[9] We will quote Sir William Blackstone's formulation:

> The duties of children to their parents arise from a principle of natural justice and retribution. For to those who gave us existence we naturally owe subjection and obedience during our minority, and honor and reverence ever after; they who protected the weakness of our infancy are entitled to our protection in the infirmity of their age; they who by sustenance and education have enabled their offspring to prosper ought in return to be supported by that offspring in case they stand in need of assistance.[10]

Christina Hoff Sommers composes a variation on this theme. She argues that the context of family life in our culture creates certain expectations that children will respect their parents. These expectations have the moral force of promises, even if the content is left vague. Sommers writes:

> In the filial situation, the basic relationship is that of nurtured to nurturer, a type of relationship that is very concrete, intimate, and long lasting, and is considered to be morally more determining than any other in shaping a variety of rights and obligations.[11]

Here again the basis for the child's obligation to care for the parent is the debt the child incurred in youth.

If the indebtedness theories sound rather calculating (I'll do this for you if you'll do that for me), the second group of theories simply denies that there is any special debt or duty incurred by the child. These might be called the I-didn't-ask-to-be-born group. In a well-known essay embodying this approach, Jane English distinguishes between favors, which must be reciprocated because they have been solicited, and voluntary sacrifices, which have not been requested and require no return. Think of the difference between asking a colleague to cover for you at work (which you can't get away with unless you are also willing to cover for her later on) and an infatuated swain who sends you a dozen roses in the hopes that you'll look with favor on his suit—which clearly leaves you with not the slightest obligation to do more than say thank you. English categorizes parental sacrifices as voluntary and concludes that if the relationship between adult children and their parents is one of friendship, it is subject to the ordinary give-and-take of favors and duties of any other friendly relation; if not, no one owes anything special to anyone.[12] Similarly, Mark

Wicclair claims children owe their parents a debt of gratitude only insofar as they value the benefits they received from them. There is no general duty of indebtedness, he says, because the child didn't contract for the goods and services the parents provided.[13] For this group of theories, there can't be a duty to care for frail parents unless the child effectively consents to it—either consents explicitly to provide the care, or at least decides that the value provided by parental sacrifices over the years was sufficiently great to invoke gratitude.

The third group of duty theories is based on gratitude even for services for which one hasn't contracted. Joel Feinberg, for one, finds a duty of gratitude that is quite different from the sort of indebtedness Blackstone describes.

> But gratitude, I submit, feels nothing at all like indebtedness. . . . My benefactor once freely offered me his services when I needed them. There was, on that occasion, nothing for me to do in return but express my deepest gratitude to him. . . . But now circumstances have arisen in which he needs help, and I am in a position to help him. Surely, I *owe* him my services now, and he would be entitled to resent my failure to come through.[14]

Jeffrey Blustein argues that gratitude is owed even where the benefactor was obliged to offer the needed services:

> It is the motive of the giver that gratitude regards, not the obligatoriness of the actions. Indeed, since the degree of obligation to gratitude is to be judged in part by how beneficial the service was to the obligated subject, and since the duties of parents are duties to protect and promote the child's serious interests, grown children may actually have more of a duty to show gratitude for benefits that were owed them than for those that were not.[15]

For both authors the duty cashes out practically, in deeds and not just sentiments.

Thinking This Over

The persistent trouble with the first group of theories—those that base duty on debt incurred in childhood—is that they don't seem to recognize that parents *owe* the children a decent minimum of the goods and services they provide. When parents fail to give children what they should, we put the children in foster care and punish the parents; it's illegal and immoral to neglect one's children. The debt-incurred theories see the relationship between parents and children as symmetrical (or, for Aristotle and Blackstone, weighted heavily in favor of the parents) but in fact, if the child is owed what the parents provide, why should the child respond with anything more than a thank you? Sommers's version is equally open to this criticism; to avoid begging the question, she would have to explain why aged parents *ought* to expect their children to look after them, and not just report that many of them do.

But the I-didn't-ask-to-be-born theories aren't very satisfactory either. If we reduce the relationship between parent and child to a simple matter of choice—if we see it as purely an *elective* affinity (to use Goethe's term), we seem to say too little. For one thing, despite birth control and abortion, many births aren't a matter of choice, and even when parents choose to have *a* child, they no more choose *this* child than it chooses them. Working out an ethics of the parent-child relationship on the basis of election and consent is a very odd thing to do, as these people didn't elect each other, nor have they consented to the relationship. For another thing, family ties differ importantly from the ties of, say, friendship or collegiality in that they persist over time through all the vicissitudes of life. You are free to allow your friendships to fade by mutual consent, but your sister is always your sister.

Family members, when it comes right down to it, **are stuck with each other.** A model of obligation based solely on affection is too contingent; we can't count on people if they have duties to us only insofar as they like us.

There's a related problem with Wicclair's claim that we have duties only insofar as we value the goods and services we receive from our parents. If a mother and father have looked after their child very well, proving themselves to be affectionate, sensible parents, the child owes them gratitude *whether or not* she values the benefits. Suppose on her birthday a cabinetmaker presented his daughter with an inlaid and delicately designed writing desk that he had made himself, only to have her remark that she doesn't really care for that sort of thing, and pass on to her next gift without thanking him. We would say of her not only that she has failed in gratitude, but that she did so because she failed to see the value of the desk and of her father's love for her. She's shown an astounding lack of moral perception.

In any case, a duty of gratitude won't help us answer the question of whether we must care for our parents, because gratitude, unlike indebtedness, can't be discharged by giving something in exchange for what was received. The daughter can't take her father out to a nice restaurant for dinner and then say to herself, "There. Now I needn't be grateful for that desk anymore." Gratitude is more like vision than like a bargain: we see, we appreciate, we are moved to thanks. This moment of seeing can occur again and again, when the daughter sits at the desk to write a letter, for example, many years after the gift was given. Blustein's account seems to be closer to the heart of the matter: gratitude, and the kinds of behavior appropriate to it, are owed to parents despite their duties to provide care. Still, the full story about duties to parents has another dimension.

The Encumbrances of Love

We see our own position on this matter as constituting a fourth kind of theory. Like the first group, we think adult children have duties of performance to their parents, but we don't base the duty in their indebtedness for goods and services received when young. Nor do we share the third group's idea that duty arises from gratitude for those services. And we certainly don't think the second group's I-didn't-ask-to-be-born argument cuts much ice. Instead, we argue that adult children's duty to care for their aged parents should be viewed in the light of another of our guiding stars: ***The need for intimacy produces responsibilities.***

As we pointed out in Chapter Two, a central function of families is to protect, nurture, and socialize their children. Parents owe their children both protection from harm and the goods of life required for human growth and development, including a reasonable amount of education. In addition to physical and educational care, though, parents also owe their children love. They must single out their children for special cherishing and affection, not only because loving and being loved is a part of a child's socialization, and not only because our biology and socialization prompt us to find our children lovable, but because the familial work of forging the child's identity is fueled by love; without it the child can't achieve either the sense of belonging to the family or the sense of separateness from the family that are essential to a sense of self. Without an abiding place in the world to be cherished and singled out specially from all others, a child is incomplete. Like Colin Turnbull's "mountain people," the Ik, she may grow up a spiritual and social cripple.[16]

The transaction that takes place between parent and young child, where the parent gives and the child receives, is in the child's case morally indeterminate. We mean that, because the child isn't yet a responsible person, he can't respond to the parents' care in a way that we can morally evaluate: it doesn't make much sense to talk of young children as either "exploiting" or "honoring" their parents, and it's not possible to attach any particular moral significance to little children's responses one way or another. We aren't claiming merely that one can't *know* what that significance is at this point; we're saying that the significance of the parent-child relationship is still being constructed. What it means now depends on what happens later. To get a clearer sense of what we mean here, consider the opening passage of James Joyce's *Portrait of the Artist as a Young Man*:

> Once upon a time and a very good time it was there was a moocow coming down the road and this moocow that was coming down along the road met a nicens little boy named baby tuckoo.... His father told him that story: his father looked at him through a glass: he had a hairy face.[17]

We attach no particular meaning to the babble about Baby Tuckoo and the hairy-faced father. That meaning is indeterminate until we are further along in the novel. Then, we may decide that Baby Tuckoo is Stephen himself, the cuckoo set in the wrong nest, and that the hairy-faced father is an image of the Roman Catholic Church, which Stephen, in a recapitulation of Lucifer's rebellion, refuses to serve. So it is with our own childhood: the full meaning of the events and relationships experienced there isn't determined until later in our life story.

When we become adults, it's one of the tasks of moral agency to sift and sort our past as we try to make sense of experience. Our family history is perhaps the greater part of the grist for this activity, for which metaphors drawn from narrative continue to be illuminating: as we reflect on our past we identify themes, select incidents, draw connections so we may create meaning for our lives. We bring into the present many of the values and virtues we acquired in childhood, but now we are free to confirm certain of them and reject others. We can do so in the choices we make—choices having to do with our education, friendships, jobs, and so on. In early adulthood we begin to plot out our life story, using the first chapter our parents wrote with us as the point of departure. That first chapter can now take on meaning as a guide to action, if we integrate the present moment of decision into the overall narrative of our lives, either by ratifying our existing course or by deliberately charting a new one. It is open to us to make our present choices in such a way as to weave our past into our future, consciously and thoughtfully constructing a meaningful moral autobiography. We described this process in Chapter Four as a nonarbitrary method of choosing among a number of morally permissible responses to illness; it can also not only shape our future, but, we believe, transfigure our past.

It can do so in this sense: parental giving and filial receiving is a major theme of the very beginning of the child's story, and there's no telling what moral significance the child will later give to it. But when he does grow into full moral adulthood, he retrospectively creates any one of a number of meanings for that theme, depending on how he treats his parents now. If his parents now come to him in need and he spurns them, he is declaring that the relationship he had with them as a child was largely instrumental: he was using them only as a means to his own ends, and they are no more to him than that. Alternatively, if he now responds to their needs, he is *redeeming* that childhood relationship of its instrumentality, and declares by his actions that he wasn't merely using his parents to provide goods and services for him.

The philosopher Christine Korsgaard has something like this idea in mind when she writes:

> You cannot, just by making a resolution, acquire a virtue or recover from a vice. Or better still, we will say that you can, because you are free, but then we must say that only what happens in the future establishes whether you have really made the resolution or not. I do not mean that only the future will produce the evidence: I mean that only what you do in the future will enable us to correctly attribute a resolution to you. There is a kind of backwards determination in the construction of one's character.[18]

Why Intimacy Isn't Merely Using People

But why shouldn't the child treat his relationship with his parents instrumentally? After all, his parents owed him care. If Jones owes Smith money and pays the debt, Smith owes him nothing in return. What's wrong with the child's taking what his parents were obliged to give and leaving it at that?

The disanalogy between Smith and the adult child lies in the fact that, oddly enough, one of the goods we give our children—our love—creates a duty on their part to love us. Parents, it will be remembered, have a duty to love their children. To discharge this particular duty, they must put themselves into a relationship of affectionate intimacy with the child—to share, to an appropriate extent, the parental self with the child. The good of love the parent gives the child isn't like food or clothing or any other object; instead, it's an emotional and psychological bond that, like other kinds of love, is incipiently mutual. The parent-child relationship in its initial stages is of course not mutual in fact, but because it's informed by love, and love seeks to be returned, it holds out the promise of reciprocity. Jones's debt to Smith is explicitly not mutual; they are on opposite sides of a fence, and when they are finished with their transaction, they are finished with each other.

Another way to put this is to say that those within a loving relationship can't remain indifferent to the needs of others within it, or else, the relationship ceases to exist. Initially this particular loving relationship is heavily one-sided, because infants' capacity to respond is limited. But as the child grows within this bond of love, he grows in awareness of the other selves that are also within the bond, for only in doing this can he get the good of love. It's a little like a conversation: I must speak as well as listen, because if I don't I have put myself outside the conversational circle. We might say that the special duty to respond to the needs of those we love is a side effect we have to accept if we are to get the good of the intimacy that is so vital to our well-being. In giving their children this relationship, parents *encumber* them, teaching them to be, not unattached, atomic individuals, but people joined to other people in many different kinds of relationships. As they live out what they are teaching, parents become vulnerable to the harm that will occur if the relationship is severed.

Consider how the harm is played out in *King Lear*. The king's mistake is not solely in confusing Cordelia's lack of ceremony with ingratitude, nor is he merely a victim of actual ingratitude at the hands of Goneril and Regan. What is "sharper than a serpent's tooth" is the thoroughgoing manner in which Goneril and Regan destroy the bonds of familial love. They continue to use the old man as means to their ends long past the dictates of necessity, refusing to acknowledge that their father, in loving them, has a legitimate reason to trust them in turn. The promise of reciprocity inherent in intimacy, fidelity, and the other goods of family life is broken, the family is sundered, the bond between parent and child betrayed. But contrary to what Sommers has written, such infidelity isn't a betrayal just because there's a widespread expectation that children will keep faith with their parents; it's a betrayal because the relationship must be encumbered with such fidelity if it is to do its job for the child in the first place. In other words, rejecting parents isn't wrong because we expect it won't happen; we expect it won't happen because it's wrong.

Those who believe that the only basis for an obligation is a contract of some kind will argue that it isn't possible to bind adults by what was done for them as children, because they were in no position to consent to the duty thrust upon them. But as we've already pointed out, human beings are forced to depend on each other to a considerable extent whether they consent to it or not, and no society could function without those who are willing to care for dependent and helpless people.[19] The loving intimacy parents owe their children requires parents to create a noninstrumental, mutual relationship. If the adult child destroys this relationship by repudiating it, he inflicts damage on them and causes them gratuitous pain.

But even if this is right, couldn't someone object that, if an adult child is without concern for his parents, it simply shows that the parents weren't successful in creating a loving relationship? If the relationship isn't there, the child can't be said to have betrayed it, and no duties follow. We think the last half of this objection is right—where there was never love but only abuse and neglect, or where bad treatment sufficiently outweighed the good to stunt whatever love might once have lain between them, the child owes no care to his parents and might even have a duty to remove himself from the situation. But the fact that no relationship exists between adult child and parent isn't proof of earlier abuse. A child might come to repudiate the relationship with his parents not because the parents didn't set up a loving one in the first place, but because of selfishness. The break could happen because the relationship didn't meet the child's standards of what love ought to be, because it became burdensome, or because it created a moral wrong greater than the wrong of repudiating the parent (for example, if the frail parent's alcoholism was endangering the adult child's relationship with other members of the family). Each of these possibilities would require its own analysis.

133

Our account of filial obligation shows that children are typically required to stay in a caring relationship with their parents. What it won't show is how and where to set limits on such care. To do that, the narrative approach we've adopted must be allowed to work in cooperation with other ethical resources, such as principles of respect for persons or various theories of social justice. Working in tandem with these, our narrative approach provides some resources for making defensible decisions about limits: it helps you make accurate judgments about whether you owe a lot or nothing at all, and it tells you why you owe what you do. We'll have more to say about how such ideas can be used to determine the limits of care in Chapter Seven.

To Get Specific

After the adult child decides *not* to repudiate the frail parent, the moral work is only just begun. What shape should the duty to the parent take? How can this duty be balanced off against other responsibilities, and what are the limits of the duty?

The answer to all these questions is, of course, "It depends." It depends on the child's life circumstances, the extent of the parent's need, whether there are other siblings in a position to help, what the parent wishes, what the siblings want, what social services and financial resources are available, to what extent it will be possible to keep the patterns of care from reinforcing oppressive stereotypes about women's work. In matters of this kind, where the particular situation varies so greatly from person to person, we again turn to Margaret Walker's idea of strong moral self-definition as a tool for of making decisions thoughtfully when faced with a welter of variables.

JEFF'S MOTHER

Jeff and Jane Morsberger, who live in San Francisco, have been married for twenty years. At first Jane worked as a legal secretary while Jeff attended law school. After he graduated it was supposed to be Jane's turn to go to school, but she found she was pregnant and, as Jeff had just been hired by a prestigious firm, she stopped work to stay home and care for the baby. Two other babies soon followed. Those years were a real struggle both financially and familially as Jeff worked to make partner and Jane looked after the children and the house.

Jeff's mother and father were divorced many years ago, when Jeff was a child. His father died when Jeff was still in law school. His mother came to live with him and Jane a few years later, after her first heart attack. Jane was very fond of the old lady and so were the children. Everyone appreciated her cooking and her effort not to disrupt the family's routines; her increasing frailty, however, soon made it impossible for her to contribute to the household as she wished.

Once the children were in school and Jeff began attracting major clients, Jane went to law school herself. Jeff felt bad about the extra amount of work she was taking on, but found his own job so demanding that he really couldn't spare time away from the office to help out on the domestic front. Somehow Jane managed to pull it all together, and now that the kids are in their teens she has a thriving general practice with a special interest in estate planning.

The years have, however, taken their toll on the marriage. Jane has often been exhausted and resentful, and Jeff has felt betrayed and angered by this. Jeff would like Jane to participate more fully in the business entertaining that is a part of his job; Jane is tired of explaining to him that someone needs to be at home in the evenings. They no longer enjoy each other very much.

Jeff's mother has become increasingly irrational, incontinent, and unpredictable, and this is creating an additional strain on the entire household. The family could afford institutional care for her, but Jeff can't forget that he told her more than once that he would never put her in a nursing home. His mother is well past the point where she could participate in any meaningful way in decisions regarding her welfare. What should Jeff do?[20]

It seems to us that Jeff faces certain constraints in his quest to respond to this crisis in an honorable way. He has a duty to remain in a relationship of intimacy with his mother; their shared history has encumbered him in ways he may not simply repudiate. But although he is alive to this consideration, he must also acknowledge the history he shares with other members of his family. He might start sorting out this tangle of values by identifying the morally important themes that have emerged in the course of his marriage, weighing them to see if he wishes to ratify or to change them. If he goes on as he has done in the past, he will perpetuate the pattern of allotting to Jane all the domestic caretaking, including the care of his mother, as long as Jane is willing to do it. He would in that case not be looking at the question of what to do for his mother from Jane's point of view, but rather would see it more abstractly, as a matter of promise-keeping or filial piety. He might also note that the burden of keeping his promise is not falling exclusively, or even equitably, on himself.

If, however, he surveyed the patterns and realized he had been considering only his own story rather than setting that story into the familial context, he might be moved to alter his course, relieving Jane of the burden of care by institutionalizing his mother, or perhaps by attempting to restructure his job so that he has more time available for attending to his mother's needs. Either way, the decision he makes is an implicit promise concerning his future conduct: he is deciding not only about a present moment, but is defining himself morally—a definition that entails a commitment to certain patterns of behavior in the future. This process of strong moral self-definition, described in the previous chapter as a means of making a nonarbitrary medical decision for oneself, also functions as we see here, when a decision must be made for another. One of its key features is the conscious recognition that the choices made in situations of this kind in a very important way determine who we are, who we have been, and who we will be as moral people; this gives the choices their proper weight, and defends us from the kind of self-deception that is sometimes a part of having to decide in morally difficult circumstances. In this application, it also invites Jeff to look at what his family is, has been, and is becoming, highlighting the relationship between his moral identity and the character of the intimate relationships in which his life is embedded.

RESPECT FOR PERSONS

"My mother still intimidates me," says fifty-eight-year-old India Wood, who is an only child. "She always had to know exactly where I was all the time, and she still does it. If I'm on the porch, she looks out the window to see what I'm doing. If I close the door to have a telephone conversation, she walks right in. She'll even walk in when I'm in the bathroom."

India's mother, now eighty-four, had been living on her own but not successfully. She was forgetful, her house was dirty, her personal hygiene was even worse, and she wasn't eating. When the strain of going back and forth each day to look after her mother began to tell on India, she persuaded the old lady to move in with her—a solution with shortcomings of its own.

The mother is dictatorial. She is sarcastic to visitors and sometimes, when India and her guests sit on the porch, the mother slams the door and locks them all out. "I'm her only child, and she doesn't like to share me," says India. "I've been divorced for a long time now, but I have five children, and whenever I was pregnant Mother would go through all the reasons why I shouldn't be. Now, when my grandchildren come to see me, Mother resents the attention I give them."

India loves to travel and once went to visit one of her children who lives in a distant city, putting her mother into a nursing home for just the week while she was away. Although India's other children came by to visit every day, the old lady made India's life so miserable on her return that she has vowed never to travel again.

"I get headaches. I worry—is this the way I'm going to be? I don't want my children to go through this. I tell them to put me in a nursing home even if I complain. I'm a good mother, so I don't feel they have to take care of me when I'm old. My mother does feel that way."[21]

As in Jeff's case, it seems India hardly needs to be reminded of the moral presumption that she should stay in the relationship with her mother. What she needs is some satisfying way of balancing her duties to her mother with a way of living that affirms her own worth as an individual. The ethical help we can offer her comes, not from the familial stars we are steering by, but rather from another constraint on action: the good old Kantian notion of respect for persons. Kant's rule is that persons must always be treated as ends in themselves, never merely as means to another person's ends. Purely instrumental uses of persons ride roughshod over something of immense moral significance about them: that they are themselves valuers and sources of value, not simply things, like cars or VCRs, which are valuable because some person finds them so. But Kant's idea of respecting persons isn't a matter of satisfying their preferences, as India is trying to do. Rather, it's a question of honoring their ability to behave morally. India, in enduring her mother's intimidating and selfish behavior, treats the old lady as if she were no longer responsible for her actions—no longer a "citizen of the kingdom of ends," to use Kant's beautiful and durable phrase. In this important respect India fails to honor her mother: she doesn't take seriously the old lady's capacity to do what's right.

India could be said to be acting out of an ethics of care, through which she responds directly and lovingly to the neediness of her mother, with whom she is in a concrete relationship. Yet an ethics of care is always vulnerable to the temptation to be disrespectful of people's moral agency. Like utilitarianism, which is based on the idea of the greatest good for the greatest number of people, an ethics of care tends to flatten out the differences among people. People become units, whether the unit be enjoyer-of-goods or cared-for, and this is to overlook the complexity of their moral lives.

People are, after all, not merely in pursuit of their own happiness but also altruistic and capable of seeing others as significant in their own right; we have inclinations and duties toward others as well as interests of our own. Charles Taylor, who has written insightfully about both our relationships to others and the individualism that seems especially to characterize the late twentieth century, invites us to go back to the historical roots of the values undergirding solidarity with others and of the values undergirding individualism, to mark and appreciate what's important about both. He thinks both are crucial, and he also thinks they aren't fully compatible with one another. The trick, then, is not to try to subsume one into the other, but rather to insist on the tension produced by bearing them both in mind simultaneously.[22] A similar strategy can be useful for sorting out the relationship between an ethics of care and of respect for the moral capacity of persons. That is, we want to be careful that, in appreciating what's good about India's love and care for her mother, we don't lose sight of how the idea of respect for persons applies to the very ill and frail as well. A distinction might be drawn between what India's mother needs and what India's mother very much desires, and what she desires may not be fully compatible with what both the mother and the daughter owe to themselves. India may well have an obligation to continue in a relationship of care with her mother; she may not have an obligation to do it on her mother's terms.

Is this paternalism? That is, aren't we encouraging India to impose on her mother India's own ideas about what's best, instead of letting India's mother decide that for herself? No. It's India's energy and time that are demanded, and India must be the judge of how to allocate them. She must distinguish between her mother's needs and wants, not "for her mother's own good," but for *India's* good.

Setting Limits

With the story of Jeff Morsberger, we suggested that attention to the family's themes can offer guidance for responding to the needs of the elderly; with the story of India Wood we examined the need to respect a person's moral capacity as well as to respond to vulnerability. But another feature these cases have in common is that they revolve around the allocation of resources within a family. It's time to tackle this issue head on. What part of the family's resources should be expended on the elderly? If the birth control pill has prevented the family from becoming unduly distended in the direction of the dependent young, what can we do to prevent the family from becoming unduly distended in the direction of the elderly? Only an overly cynical view of the family would deny there is a duty to care for the aged; only an overly romantic view would deny there are limits to such care.

When these intergenerational dynamics are put in the context of modern medicine, setting limits becomes a social problem as well as a familial one. This is so because many of the resources that are at issue here are social ones and because setting proper limits increasingly seems to require some shared idea of what constitutes both a good life and a good death. If, for example, we as a society hold the view that death is a disease to be conquered and old age a wild frontier whose boundaries we must never cease to beat back, we will continue to expend resources on expensive, high-technology health care for the very old. We will devote many research dollars to extending life as long as possible, and insist that our grandparents not only be offered but also coaxed to accept burdensome therapeutic regimens so long as any hope of life remains.

If, on the other hand, we consider old age a fitting and natural close to the human lifespan, with its own rhythms and its own rightful place in the scheme of things, and if we consider that those who have lived to the age of seventy or more have likely been able to experience what the philosopher Norman Daniels calls the "normal opportunity range" for our society, we might think it proper to ask the old to yield a little to the young.[23] We might, for example, reach agreement that the resources expended on a costly liver transplant for an eighty-year-old would be better spent on education, and we might agree that we are socially obligated to construct the economic mechanisms that would allow this transfer of resources to take place. To appreciate this point one need only consider the contrast between an urban hospital's intensive care unit, where the old lie waiting to die for weeks or even months at staggering cost, and the inner-city elementary school in the next block, where six-year-olds are crammed forty to a classroom—perhaps a windowless classroom—and even the out-of-date textbooks must be shared because the school is badly underfunded.[24]

"What kind of sense can we make of old age, of the fact that our bodies change and decline, sicken and decay, and then die?" This question, posed by the philosopher Daniel Callahan in his book *Setting Limits*, is one that we, both as a society and within our families, can no longer afford to evade.

> If the aged are to understand themselves, and if our society is to make sense of them in their increased numbers and growing demand on resources, then the meaning and significance of old age must be a matter of open discussion and of an effort to shape some social agreement.[25]

How can this be done? Callahan proposes a balance of the new possibilities the late twentieth century offers the elderly, with the traditional and valuable idea that old age is a time for wise but not supine withdrawal from the affairs of this world. The notion that life should be divided into "stages" which come complete with their own complement of appropriate activities may seem—at least if we are speaking of adults—to be offensive, oppressive, and reactionary. It conjures up images of pre-Enlightenment societies, ruled by the metaphor of the Great Chain of Being, of the medieval Christian knight fighting in youth for honor and the glory of God, but in old age retiring to a monastery to contemplate his death and the life to come. Such heavily laden metaphors and roles aren't available to us anymore, and perhaps that's all to the good. But at the same time, some significant common themes do run through the experiences of old people. If our limited social resources suggest the need to start living our lives with greater attention to how they affect others, those common themes may provide some clues to a broadly outlined, flexible concept of what it is to age with personal dignity and respect for the common weal.

Oddly enough, it's not so much medicine's power but medicine's uncertainty that tends to pull against the measured view of death. As things stand, medicine isn't able to "cure" mortality, or even extend the human lifespan sufficiently to cause us to alter longstanding intuitions about what it is to be old. Many more people live to eighty-five now than did in the 1890s, but to be eighty-five is still to be old, and there is not much reason to think any medical alchemy will be able to transmute eight decades of life into youth, or even into vigorous middle age. What medicine can do is continually apply pressure against the process of aging, at least so long as any uncertainty remains about the outcome of a given intervention for a given condition. If an elderly patient is admitted to the hospital with a treatable problem, the health care team will treat it, and then treat the next problem, and the next, all the while unsure whether the process of systemic bodily shutdown is reversible or whether it will lead to the patient's death. By the time certainty about this can be achieved, the patient will have undergone intensive treatment, some of it intended to cure, and the rest to provide palliative care. It is this steady escalation of treatment under uncertainty that is responsible for the fact that almost thirty percent of the Medicare money any one person will use in her old age is spent in the last year of her life.[26] And that's only Medicare money. In 1987, when the elderly represented twelve percent of the population, they accounted for thirty-six percent of total personal health care expenditures, averaging $5,360 per year as compared to $1,290 per year for younger persons; about a fourth of the average expenditure came not from Medicare but from direct payments by or for the old person.[27]

Our prevalent social attitude about mortality, if medical practice is any accurate reflection, seems to be that it's all right to die—but not *of* anything. Is this attitude appropriate? Is it consistent with the best understanding of our deepest social values, and our most pressing human needs? Can our society afford to keep spending this kind of money on the last years of life? Should families keep insisting that the doctors "do everything" for their very old?

While it would be vulgar to reduce to economics our social and individual attempts to forge a sense of what it means to live and die, money is not irrelevant. For example, a study followed 146 patients who were given cardiopulmonary resuscitation (CPR) after suffering cardiac arrest while they were already in the hospital. The study showed that while eighty-four of the patients were revived, only seven patients, or five percent, lived long enough to leave the hospital. The cost of attempting CPR on the eighty-four patients was $1.1 million, and because that produced a gain of only seven lives saved, the cost of CPR in that particular hospital is $150,000 per survivor. A similar study looked at one hundred and fifty patients who were critically ill with cancer. Those who spent time in the intensive care unit for any reason other than postoperative recovery were treated at a cost of between $82,845 and $189,339 for every year of life gained.[28]

A fundamental idea here is finitude, and a proper appreciation of finitude must reflect awareness of the finite resources our communities have to make a good life for all their citizens. Our efforts to combat the finitude of the human lifespan are greatly weakening our ability to respond to other needs. For every American car now on the market, for example, an average of roughly $800 of the sticker price reflects the cost of the autoworkers' health insurance. This $800 is in effect a kind of tax on the car, directed at one small segment of the population (car-buyers) for one very specific purpose (health care), using up resources that can't then be directed toward investment in industry, nor for subsidizing the fine arts, nor toward providing housing for those in need, nor for education, nor for improved public transportation, nor for any other thing worth having. And while the consumer subsidizes the autoworker's health insurance in this way, thirty-eight million other Americans go without insurance altogether.

What can families do about this? Let's look at one family's actual experience and see what we can learn from it.

HELGA WANGLIE'S VENTILATOR

On 14 December 1989 Helga Wanglie, eighty-six, broke her hip when she slipped on a rug in her home in Minneapolis. By the first of January she had developed respiratory failure, so she was put on a ventilator. Over the next five months, the staff of the Hennepin County Medical Center repeatedly tried to wean her from it, but without success. At this point Mrs. Wanglie was conscious, able to acknowledge pain, and aware of her family. She was transferred to a facility that specializes in the care of ventilator-dependent patients. On 23 May 1990 her heart stopped and she stopped breathing. She was resuscitated and transferred to a hospital in St. Paul, but it was determined that she had suffered extremely severe and irreversible brain damage. The St. Paul hospital's ethics committee reviewed her case and doctors discussed with the family the possibility of limiting further life-sustaining treatment, but the immediate family—her husband, daughter, and son—resisted this idea and requested that she be transferred back to Hennepin County, where they felt she had received excellent care.

She was readmitted there on 31 May 1990 and treated vigorously with continued ventilator support, antibiotics for recurrent pneumonia, artificial feeding, and treatment for electrolyte and fluid imbalance. Over the next several months, repeated evaluations by the neurology and pulmonary medicine services confirmed the diagnosis of persistent vegetative state and permanent respirator dependency because of chronic lung disease. The medical staff viewed Mrs. Wanglie's prognosis as extremely poor, and didn't believe that the ventilator could benefit her. However, her family insisted that all forms of treatment be continued.

Oliver Wanglie understood that his wife was unaware of herself, her surroundings, and his visits. When asked if he understood that there is no recovery from a persistent vegetative state and that Mrs. Wanglie could never improve in any significant way, he replied, "That may be true, but we hope for the best." His view was that only God can take life and that doctors should not play God.

By late 1990 it became apparent that the conflict between the family's insistence on continued medical treatment and the hospital staff's strong feelings that further treatment was futile could not be resolved. The hospital filed papers seeking appointment of a conservator other than Mr. Wanglie to decide whether continued treatment was appropriate. The case—the first in the United States in which a hospital sought a conservator to consider nontreatment when the immediate family strongly and unanimously objected—was heard on 28 May 1991, and ended in a ruling that Mr. Wanglie was fully competent to continue as his wife's decision-maker. Mrs. Wanglie died on 4 July 1991.

The cost of Mrs. Wanglie's care at Hennepin County Medical Center alone was over $800,000. The entire amount was paid by the Wanglie's health maintenance organization and by a private supplementary insurance plan.[29]

When a family member falls into a persistent vegetative state—a state in which the person lies permanently beyond pain, beyond dreaming, beyond thoughts or experiences, beyond anything that could count as meaningful in human life—the family must ask itself what it expects medicine to do here. Cure or improvement are not possible; with great care the organic systems can be preserved and that is all. Was Mr. Wanglie enlisting medicine's help while he waited for God to perform a miracle? But surely if God were so inclined, He could perform the miracle even if the ventilator were shut off. Did Mr. Wanglie think that, as money was no object for him, and he lived in a society that allows the rich to buy all the luxuries they can afford he was free to purchase whatever he wanted? But health care is not the same sort of commodity as a yacht or a Porsche; for one thing, other people in the Wanglie's health maintenance organization and other subscribers to the supplementary insurance plan were subsidizing Mrs. Wanglie's care, and for another, some basic minimum of health care is necessary to everyone, although Porsches and yachts are not. Health care must be used responsibly or there will not be enough to go around.

Or was Mr. Wanglie simply giving voice to his wife's conviction of the immense moral significance of organic human life plain and simple? From the perspective of the Wanglie family, perhaps Mrs. Wanglie was not for all intents and purposes dead, the recipient of useless, extremely expensive care, but rather merely massively and tragically handicapped, yet still alive, with a life as significant as the life of any other human being.

The Wanglie case points out how a family's value system can come into sharp conflict with an emerging theme in medical ethics—the idea that, far from having an obligation to sustain life as long as possible, medicine is under no obligation to provide "futile" care, where "futile" means not capable of achieving what medicine regards as being of any benefit: similar conflicts have been reported in neonatal intensive care units, where it seems that it's no longer so common for aggressive doctors to force care on extremely ill infants over the protestations of family, but rather for doctors to feel that children should be allowed to die, while their families are still clamoring for every possible intervention. Nancy M. P. King has pointed out how these conflicting points of view often result from a lack of continual communication between health care providers and the family; the health care team forms a gradual consensus about what should be done through conversations the family isn't a part of, and so the family takes much longer to arrive at the caregivers' conclusions. If discussion about the development of the case were more open to the family, there might be fewer disagreements.[30]

But disagreements may at base not be merely a matter of bad communication or timing; there may be a clash of significantly different values. A family in the Wanglies' situation can be guided by considerations of justice and moderation, but they might also exercise the principle of respect for persons we alluded to above, whereby they suppose that Mrs. Wanglie would not have wanted to take more than her fair share of medical help. Despite our regard for human life, people do not generally believe that any given individual has a right to unlimited resources in order to avoid death. So the Wanglie family might, in allowing the ventilator to be withdrawn, honor by proxy Mrs. Wanglie's status as a moral agent. Families like the Wanglies can, while remaining faithful to their relationships, steer by one of our familial stars, distinguishing between love for the family member and the insistence that doctors "do everything." They aren't abandoning the patient even though they decline certain medical interventions; after all, *In families, motives matter a lot.*

All that being said, it's important to point out that, by the terms of their insurance agreements, the Wanglies had a strong case for saying that they weren't taking more than their fair share of resources; everything was done in service of a goal they found of great importance. To mediate this kind of dispute between families and medicine, we need the support of the wider society. If, for example, there were broad social agreement that ventilators are an inappropriate treatment for patients in the persistent vegetative state, and if hospitals had clear regulations to this effect, the weight of the decision would lie not with Mr. Wanglie individually, nor with health care professionals determining what kind of life is worth how much health care, but with all of us collectively—as is proper for decisions about social policy.[31] Cases like this show that decisions about how the health care system should be reorganized, directed, and focused may require that we as a society come to a rather detailed consensus concerning human life, other human goods, and the economic means to pursue them. Moreover, we'll have to give thought to those individuals and families whose traditions and values lie outside that consensus.

Chapter Five

PUT MOM WITH THE DEMENTED?

In a first-rate home for the aged lives seventy-eight-year-old Marìa Lopez, badly demented due to Alzheimer's disease. Mrs. Lopez's daughter Carmelita, with whom she had lived since she was widowed twenty-five years previously, was forced to admit her mother to the facility about a year ago when she was no longer able to care for her at home. Carmelita Lopez now lives alone, but comes to see her mother almost every day on her way home from work. Because she was convinced her mother would have hated it, she didn't have her admitted to Floor Three, where the other severely demented residents live. But in recent weeks Mrs. Lopez's behavior has become so disruptive that the staff have been receiving complaints from the other patients on her floor.

The psychiatrist has proposed psychotropic medication, but Carmelita Lopez has rejected that suggestion even more vigorously than the proposal to move her mother: she says Marìa, always a very sociable, outgoing woman, must not be put on drugs that would remove all possibility of interaction with other people. She understands that the situation is hard on her mother's neighbors but hopes they will be decent about it; she simply can't permit them to put her mother among senile people whose company would have been so very uncongenial to her.

If families like the Wanglies put into stark relief the problem of setting limits on extremely expensive end-of-life care, families like the Lopezes must be encouraged to set limits of a different kind: limits on the amount of neighborliness they demand of others. What would ideally be best for Mrs. Lopez under the theory of substituted judgment (which is what her daughter is employing) is clearly a hardship to the community in which the old lady lives. To insist on what her mother would have wished even when the wish may be harming others is to lose sight of every consideration other than the preferences of the patient.

In any case, it's not clear that Carmelita Lopez is an accurate reporter. She couches her concerns in terms of what her mother would have wanted, but a closer look reveals that what's importantly at issue is Carmelita's own need for her mother, who is the only family she has. The reason she gives for refusing the psychotropic medication makes it plain that she has not yet fully assimilated the fact of her mother's severe dementia; the

Alzheimer's disease removed all possibility of interaction with other people some time ago, but Carmelita needs this facet of her mother's personality so badly that she behaves as if there were still hope of it reappearing. When families lay claim to resources whose cost to others is unreasonably high, they must examine the possibility that they are doing so out of their own needs or feelings of guilt, and not because the patient is justly entitled to those resources. These needs and feelings must be acknowledged and, where possible, alleviated, but it is better for all concerned if they are not unwittingly used to fuel immoderate demands on the health care delivery system.

WHEN THE STAFF BECOMES THE FAMILY

How does one negotiate limits to care when the patient has been in the nursing home for so long that the primary care providers have "adopted" him? Lars Nielsen, an eighty-one-year-old farmer, was admitted to the Maple Grove Home in southeastern South Dakota two years ago, after having been hospitalized for a stroke. When he entered the home he was ambulatory but unable to care for himself in any way, and incapable of speech. Some months later he developed pneumonia, and after prolonged bedrest lost his ability to walk. Further bouts of pneumonia were complicated by congestive heart failure.

Mr. Nielsen then stopped eating, so the staff considered a nasogastric tube. When his wife was informed of this she wrote a letter explaining that her husband wouldn't want to be fed in this way. Because Mr. Nielsen could still be fed by syringe, the idea of the feeding tube was dropped; but, as the staff had some doubts about how closely Mrs. Nielsen's letter actually reflected her husband's wishes, corroborating statements were obtained from Mr. Nielsen's brother and two of his friends. During this period Mrs. Nielsen, who suffers from arthritis, no longer visited her husband as frequently as before, and she no longer phoned the nursing home as often to inquire about him. The nursing staff took this as not only an abandonment of Mr. Nielsen but also of them.

Six weeks later even the syringe feedings failed, but no feeding tube was inserted. As four and then five days went by during which Mr. Nielsen ate nothing at all, it became obvious that the nursing staff was finding it very difficult to watch their patient die. "We're his family now," remarked one of the nurse's aides bitterly, "but all we can do is stand by while Mrs. Nielsen starves her husband to death."[32]

Nursing homes are unlike hospitals in the length of time caregivers have to grow fond of their patients. Their doing so is a natural and human response, and perhaps none of us would want to be nursed by anyone who was incapable of caring *about* us as well as *for* us. It's all the more important, then, that caregivers understand and respect the difference between fondness and familial intimacy. It was in the bosom of his family, many years ago, that Mr. Nielsen's self was forged, and it was within the family he later created with his wife that his self was maintained and continued to grow. It is she who knows him best; she whose investment in a lifetime of living with him and concern for him entitles her to speak for him now. The nursing staff have had nothing to do with his process of self-maintenance. Indeed, by the time Mr. Nielsen came to the nursing home, he was no longer capable of forming relationships with anyone, and certainly not relationships in which his self would continue to be forged.

Where does the self go when, as with Mr. Nielsen, it seems to recede in the face of a stroke or dementia? If it goes anywhere at all, surely it goes into the people to whom Mr. Nielsen has been closest over the years—to the people who remember him in his vigor and have loved him longest.[33] The nursing staff presumes too much when they think of themselves as his "family," for *he* has never entered into a relationship with *them* at all, even if they are fond of him. The relationship is too one-sided to count as the sort of intimacy these caregivers are claiming. Any number of things could be preventing Mrs. Nielsen from attending daily at her husband's bedside; she is in frail health herself, and she knows he is past understanding whether she is there.

It will be increasingly important in the coming years for long-term care facilities to teach their staffs about the ethics of end-of-life decision-making. Caregivers in nursing homes are often poorly educated and badly underpaid; they do difficult work under very trying conditions. If no one troubles to assuage their outraged feelings or helps them to navigate troubling deathbed scenarios, their work is made even more difficult than it has to be.

Negotiating With Death

The question of a "good death" is a particularly vexing one, given the natural tendency to deny and fear death, and to put it off for as long as possible. Because medical technology allows us to do it and because the American attitude is, "Don't just stand there—do something!" more deaths are being negotiated rather than merely suffered; the clinical ethicist and lawyer Nancy Dubler predicts it will soon be as many as two out of three.[34]

The Wanglie case illustrates the desire to postpone the final moment at all costs, but there is the opposite response to death, which is to get it over with while one is still in charge of one's faculties. If the nursing home staff caring for Lars Nielsen must be taught to adjust to the realities of negotiated death, so must we all. If death can be negotiated once the dying process nears its end, we will be tempted to negotiate it at an earlier stage—through euthanasia and assisted suicide. Achieving some kind of social consensus about the legitimacy of this sort of negotiation has become a pressing problem.

Is suicide morally justifiable under some circumstances, and if so, don't those same circumstances justify assisting someone to commit suicide? Is it ever all right to take an innocent person's life, even with the person's consent? If it's all right for others to do this, mightn't we still want physicians—who already have such power over life and death and to whom we are already so vulnerable—to refrain from such killing?

The proper role of physicians at the end of life is hotly contested. Impassioned arguments in favor of allowing doctors to assist in their patients' suicides collide with equally impassioned arguments insisting doctors must not kill. We feel the attraction of both sets of arguments, but the issue is too complex to sort out here. We're going to have to restrict ourselves to the perplexities facing family members who don't know what to do as their loved ones die.[35]

An ethics of the family should help untangle these perplexities. It's useful to think about how *Family members are stuck with each other,* that *Families are ongoing stories,* and how *Family members aren't replaceable by similarly (or better) qualified people* as we sort out what it means actively to end one's life.

Chapter Five
WITH HIS BOOTS ON

Tecumseh Smith lived on a Cherokee reservation in western Oklahoma. The land is poor; from the time when the Cherokee were thrust out of Georgia over a century ago to walk the Trail of Tears, the tribe has been driven onto land no one else wanted. When oil was discovered in Cherokee territory in Oklahoma the people were forced to move again, and now the reservations are far from the derricks and the industries that produce wealth for European Americans.

Tecumseh Smith attained his biblical threescore years and ten without once setting foot off the reservation. Poverty and drunkenness were his constant companions, as were his love for his son, the "boys" with whom he hunted and fished, and the land he roamed. Although his liver was hardening it still functioned after a fashion, which was more than could be said for the Islets of Langerhans in his pancreas. Years of alcoholism and a genetic predisposition had produced adult-onset diabetes, now so far out of control that his right foot became gangrenous. Medical measures to save it were unsuccessful, and his doctors told him he would die unless his foot were amputated at once.

"I can't be bothered with it," declared Tecumseh Smith. "Me'n the boys are going out in my son's pickup truck tomorrow to shoot rabbits."

His son, who had brought him to the clinic, exchanged anxious glances with the doctor. "Can't do it, Pa. The truck's got a busted axle."

"First I heard of it. How about my fishing rod—that got a busted axle too? If I can't hunt I can still gimp over to the river and pull the catfish out."

"I don't think you understand, Pa. You can't put it off. You'll be dead within the month if you don't let them take that foot. Now. Today. Isn't that right, Dr. Gupta?"

Dr. Gupta nodded.

"I hear you." Tecumseh Smith said nothing more. Instead, he picked up his crutches and swung himself furiously out of the clinic and into the parking lot. When his son caught up with him the old man would not speak to him, but hobbled on until he reached his trailer. There he pulled down his rifle and a box of shells, and threw into an old knapsack some canned goods, matches, a change of clothing, a bottle of whiskey, and his hunting knife.

"Where you going, Pa?"

"I'm going up country, same as my ancestors did. Saw it in a movie once.

When your time's up, it's up—no sense in fooling around. I'm going to have me one last good rabbit-shoot—good's I can get it on crutches, anyway—and then I'm dying with my boots on. And I don't want no company."

The old man died three days later in a diabetic coma, in a camp he had made for himself some five miles north of the settlement. His son found him there and brought him home for burial. He did not remove his boots.

Middle-class and wealthy Americans have a wide range of choices available to them; their general approach to life is to negotiate among these choices to their best advantage. The poor find it harder to see life as a matter of making the best bargains one can; the circumstances of life are often simply what one is stuck with. The strength of this last insight lies in reminding us of the natural limits of existence—it shows us that we are finite human creatures and not gods after all. The danger of the insight is that it can become a temptation to passivity and fatalism, lulling us into a premature acceptance of death when reasonable measures for preserving life are still available. Mr. Smith acquiesced to his death because the alternative would leave him permanently unable to engage in the hunting and fishing that were so important to him; his son perhaps thought he had given up too soon. These judgments are intensely personal, yet when we try to decide whether Mr. Smith's acceptance of death was wise, we might also try to see life as he did, as something other than a playing-field for the free and unfettered will.

Is any of this his son's business? Of course. The young man cares about his father, loves him, is concerned for him. And the old man loves his son. That relationship gives the son the right to be involved in the decision: the old man owes him the explanation he provided, and the young man owes his father the attempt to determine if the old man understands what's at stake. The son may even try to get his father to change his mind. But what both parties must do, after they try to understand each other, is to acknowledge that the decision ultimately belongs to the father. It is his own life and not the son's that is at stake, his own integrity he is trying to preserve.

We can, however, imagine situations in which a family member legitimately has a far greater say than Tecumseh Smith's son over what is to be done, even where the patient disagrees with the treatment proposed. This can be so even when the treatment interferes with the patient's plan for a good death. A final story:

Chapter Five

THE PHARMACIST'S WIFE

Kezia and Vernon Whatley have been married for forty years. Like other black families in LaGrange, Alabama, the Whatleys have known economic hardship, but they managed to feed, clothe, and educate their three children, all of whom now live in the North with families of their own. Kezia has been the office manager at a cable TV company for the last ten years, and Vernon is a pharmacist employed by a large drugstore chain.

Kezia is dying of ovarian cancer. Radiation therapy can no longer help her, nor, really, can any other form of "comfort" care. She lies in her bed with a large open sore in her belly that stinks foully. The stench is so bad she's ashamed to have anybody in the same room with her; she kept apologizing to her children and grandchildren when they recently came to see her. Her pain is excruciating, yet the only way it can be controlled now is by doping her into unconsciousness. The indignity and the physical agony have become intolerable, and today Kezia has decided to put an end to it.

"You've got to help me, Vern. You know what drugs to give me so it'll be quick and easy. I can't stand this any more. Please, please give me something that'll kill me."

Vernon has seen this coming for days, and has spent many sleepless hours agonizing over it. He's thought about talking to his minister about it, but knows the minister will tell him to leave it to the Lord. "It's not that you won't be troubled, it's not that you'll see your way easily," he preached recently, "but when you are in darkness and doubt, hang on to Jesus and obey the Ten Commandments and you'll come safe through the valley to the other side."

He tells his wife he can't do it—that it's an evil thing to kill. Kezia pleads with him, begging him to stop her suffering and then, as he still refuses, accusing him of keeping his conscience clean at her expense. The accusation wounds Vernon deeply, and for the time being no more is said.

Later in the day, when Kezia is momentarily lucid and again begs him to help her, he takes her hand in his and sadly shakes his head. "I'll do anything for you I can," he says, "but I can't give away my soul. When I stand before God that's all I've got, and I can't give it up even for you."

Painful scenes of this kind may well become more common as the public debate over euthanasia and assisted suicide gains momentum. The idea of ending one's life in the face of unbearable suffering seems less repugnant than it did in the days when suicides were buried outside the churchyard. But whatever conclusions one reaches regarding the ethics of such an act, one would be hard put to it to defend the idea that a person has a duty to act contrary to his conscience. Vernon Whatley has considered the matter carefully and concluded that he must not help his wife to kill herself. He has a stake in the matter: he is being asked to violate his own integrity as best he understands it. Because the stake is so high he is justified in refusing to help, even though his refusal is contrary to the patient's wishes and the stakes for her are life and death.

We would argue that a family member may refuse other kinds of help, too, even when a good death for the patient is at stake. Suppose a woman is dying of breast cancer. There is an outside possibility that an autologous bone marrow transplant might give her five more years of life, but, because the therapy has not so far been demonstrated to be beneficial, her insurance company won't pay for the transplant. Has her family wronged her if it doesn't provide the necessary money? Not if doing so would seriously compromise its ability to meet its major responsibilities. Other family members also have a claim on these financial resources. For that reason, the patient may not demand the lion's share of them, even when she is dying.

Decisions of this kind are not easy; they never should be. It's hard to think of any rule—even in the law—that can keep us from ever making a mistake. And while the law often expresses our society's moral understandings, it sometimes gets things wrong; it might turn out occasionally that if one is to do the right thing, one must break the law to do it. Mercy, compassion, love, and respect might all compel a person to civil disobedience in the form of assisting a family member's suicide. To say no to this wife or son when their need is so great might sometimes be an act of moral abandonment even more serious than breaking a law. If we try to play it safe, assuming that patient preference should always be our guide, or else assuming that we must always obey the social rule against killing the innocent, we are occasionally going to make a very serious mistake indeed.

Let us be clear about this. It will sometimes turn out that the moral thing for a family member to do is to kill or assist in the suicide of a dying loved one. To hold otherwise is to say that everyone has a duty to live, and not just a right to life. While life is indeed precious, so too is a person's sense of her own dignity, so too is relief from torture. Those who love the dying person sometimes hold all these precious things in their keeping and must choose among them. This choice is perhaps best guided by careful attention to the circumstance of the dying person, the circumstance of the person whose aid is enlisted, and the character of the story that binds the two together.

The kind of aid family members will most often need to provide, however, is not lethal. It is the comfort of their companionship, their love and care. And more even than this, it is the capacity of the family to become the primary repository of the memory of the person once death has occurred. The person within a family belongs, after all, to an ongoing story which he plays a particular and irreplaceable part in creating. That is no bad thing to leave behind.

Chapter Six

When Medicine Makes Babies

MEDICINE'S MOST DRAMATIC IMPACT ON THE FAMILY HAS PROBABLY
been in the area of assisted reproduction. Here medical technology and the
desire to help the subfertile have combined to reconfigure, radically, our
understanding of what constitutes a family. Assisted reproduction
produces new and distinctly odd kinship patterns: a child's older brother
can be his fraternal twin, thanks to frozen embryo technology, and a
woman can be genetically related to her child without ever having given
birth, thanks to implant technology. But because the new technologies
reinforce only certain features of families and not others, they also subtly
reinforce troubling ideas about how family members ought to feel and
behave toward each other. Such medical technology, with its windows into
wombs and its tests for previously occult genetic disorders, introduces a
degree of "quality control" into our selection of our children unknown in
human history. Medicine's solutions to subfertility, quality control over
babies, and ability to manipulate genetic matter reveal its misunderstand-
ing of both familial values and familial vulnerabilities.

Conversely, the pressure families put on medicine to help out when the old-fashioned method of having babies isn't working has had wide-ranging consequences for health care. To what extent should medicine succumb to familial pleas for pregnancy? Is subfertility an illness? Traditionally, medicine's goals have been to heal and relieve suffering caused by sickness. If the profession can be seduced into satisfying the desire to form and tailor families, what is to stop it from medicalizing just any sort of problem to which it can offer a solution? Medicine's ambitions are already overweening. Familial pressures only serve to distort further its already distorted self-understanding.

Subfertility is a painful experience, as anyone who has repeatedly tried and failed to have children can tell you. Of married couples in this country who want to have children (government statistics aren't available for the unmarried), 8.5 percent cannot, either because of a low sperm count, blocked fallopian tubes, lack of a uterus, or some other condition.[1] The traditional solution to this problem—adoption—has become increasingly difficult. Single parents are apt to be allowed to adopt only handicapped or older children, which may not be at all what they had in mind. Even the two million traditionally married couples in the U.S. who are subfertile far outnumber the country's 365,000 orphans: if each couple adopted one orphan, that would still leave 1,635,000 couples without a child.[2] Some people travel to countries where adoptable children are more abundant, but this can involve prolonged stays and the payment of high fees to the parties arranging the adoption.

In any case, many subfertile people experience a strong desire to bring into being the children they rear. For them, adoption is distressingly inadequate. They may feel that the bond between parent and child is deepened if there is a biological link as well as a social one, or they may simply feel shame at the inability to do something as natural as producing a baby. For some people, the urge to reproduce oneself relates in some way to the desire to survive one's death; for others, the instinct is closer to the artist's urge to make something that will outlast its creator's lifetime.[3]

A TALE OF TWO SISTERS

These rather metaphysical considerations aren't the only reasons people want to have children of their own bodies. Other motives are intensely practical. In April of 1990, for example, Mary and Abe Ayala, of Walnut, California, had a baby to provide bone marrow for their seventeen-year-old daughter Anissa, dying of chronic myelogenous leukemia. The baby, Marissa, stood a one-in-four chance of having bone marrow that matched her sister's; she turned out to be compatible.

When she was fourteen months old, Marissa was anesthetized so that a surgeon could insert an inch-long needle into her hip and slowly begin to withdraw bone marrow. After removing a cupful of the red liquid, the medical team carried it to another room where Anissa lay waiting, her own diseased bone marrow having been killed by intensive doses of radiation and chemotherapy administered twelve days earlier. A physician began feeding the baby's bone marrow into a Hickman catheter inserted in Anissa's chest.

And then came the long wait. Anissa's body might have rejected the bone marrow cells or, because the chemotherapy left her immunosuppressed, she might have picked up a fatal infection. But doctors rated the chance of success at seventy percent, and events proved them right. In June of 1992, Anissa, now twenty years old and completely free of leukemia, was married to Bryan Espinosa at a historic mansion in Redlands, California. Her little sister Marissa was the flower girl.[4]

Was it wrong to have a child so its bone marrow could be harvested? Doesn't this violate the Kantian maxim that one must never treat others solely as a means to one's own ends? In the previous chapter we argued that the instrumentality of childhood can't be given moral significance until we see how the grown child responds to his own parents' needs. Similarly, the instrumentality of Marissa's conception doesn't take on much moral force until we see how the family feels about and behaves toward the child. We can't say whether it was right or wrong to conceive her until we know how she is treated. Marissa now seems, however, to be having a good life, with loving parents and older siblings who care for her and have welcomed her into the family.

Consider what might have happened instead. A few years ago when a young boy in the western United States was slowly dying of a genetic disease, physicians told his parents what the Ayalas were told—that if he could have a perfectly matched bone marrow transplant his disease might be cured. But he was an only child, so his parents also decided to conceive a bone marrow donor. In this case, however, the baby, whose bone marrow was successfully transplanted into its older brother, was given away by its parents. They put it up for adoption.[5] These parents could not have said more clearly that the child had been conceived only for its bone marrow, and that their relationship to it was to be purely instrumental. By contrast, the Ayalas, in caring for and welcoming Marissa, have redeemed their relationship of its initial instrumentality and honored the child as a person in her own right.

In Families, Motives Matter: it makes a difference whether you start a pregnancy because you want a sister for little Johnny, or because you hope a baby will hold your marriage together, or because you believe women are simply unfulfilled unless they procreate. On the other hand, there would seem to be very few single moments—including the moment of conception—whose motives are capable of defining the moral quality of an intimate relationship: this must unfold gradually, over time, in an ongoing story.

What Parents Owe Their Children

Why does producing a baby for its marrow and then giving it up for adoption strike us as heartless? Where do our duties to care for our children come from, anyway? Here, as with filial duties of care for one's parents, the obligation doesn't seem to be grounded in consent. It's *Causing someone to exist* that *produces responsibilities.*

Let's run over the reasoning for this star again and see how far we can extend it. When I cause a child to exist I am obliged to look after it, not because I have consented to impregnate the birthgiver, nor because I have chosen not to have an abortion, nor merely because there is a social contract to the effect that parents must rear their own children.[6] Rather, I am responsible for the child's care because in the process of bringing her into existence I have put her life at risk. I can't help doing this—it's what any human baby faces. A baby, after all, is a helpless little person who is so vulnerable that it will die without care. Because I've helped bring about this person's predicament, I have a duty to look after her until she is old enough to look after herself; I'm obliged to get her out of the danger I've gotten her into. Looked at in this way, procreation is a little like running someone over in one's car. Even if the driver didn't intend to harm the person she hit, she can't just drive off. Where we create a vulnerability we have, a responsibility to stand by the victim.

To push this analogy, when you hit someone with your car you make an existing person worse off than he was before. By contrast, bringing a baby into the world doesn't make it worse off, because if you hadn't conceived it, it wouldn't exist at all. By this reasoning, the child who was conceived for its bone marrow and then given up for adoption has no cause for complaint: if his bone marrow hadn't been wanted he would never even have been born.

But let's try the same reasoning in another situation. Pretend, for a moment, that there is a subfertile woman who can conceive only if she takes a certain drug, Concepticon. Suppose, further, that one of the side-effects of Concepticon, is that, when the child who is born with its help reaches the age of eighteen, he will contract a hideous disease unless he is provided with an antidote that the Concepticon Company manufactures. Is there any doubt that the company has a duty to keep manufacturing the antidote? Concepticon didn't make the child worse off than he would have been if he'd never been born—in fact, without the drug, he never *would* have been born—but because the company is responsible for the latent disease that accompanies his existence, we would find it reprehensible if it shut down its antidote operations and left the child to suffer.

The Concepticon example indicates that causing a predicament entails at least some responsibility for extricating the person from it. But suppose there were other manufacturers of the Concepticon antidote. Can't the company fulfill its responsibility by making sure other mechanisms are in place to meet the child's needs? Possibly, so long as it stands by in case the mechanisms fail. Then didn't the parents of the marrow donor fulfill their responsibility by finding other caregivers who were willing to adopt the child? Well, no. One difference between businesses and families is that *Family members aren't replaceable by similarly (or better) qualified people.* Why? Because the work of the family is quite different from merely seeing that certain commodities are available for those who need them. Anybody can deliver a commodity, but the functions of families are complex, multi-faceted, personal, and particular. Families are structures of intimacy in which children first and most fundamentally develop their identities; those identities have something to do with who the particular people are who share the child's history. When someone remarks to a child, "You're just like your grandmother," the child has a vivid sense of how she fits into the world, and that other identifiable people are like her in certain ways. In this respect, that particular grandmother is not replaceable by other grand-mothers. At birth the child has already come to have a place within the family's story—a heritage, a role in the scheme of things. Necessity might dictate that she lose this place and occupy another within a different family, but she has then lost something that was uniquely her own.

Furthermore, the point isn't really whether someone else would do as good a job at rearing a child; it's that it's *the parent's* job. A parent on the scene is in a position to continually monitor his own efforts with respect to the child's well-being. He can't do this for a substitute parent, especially if he removes himself from daily involvement in the child's life. His relation-ship to the agency of others is categorically different from his relationship to his own agency: he can only predict that someone else will meet the child's needs, but he can guarantee, within the limits of what's possible, that he'll do it himself.

Even if he knows the proposed replacement-parent very well, he can't insure that proper care will be given. Serious disagreements as to what constitutes appropriate treatment of children often break out between adults who have had a great deal of opportunity to get to know one another over a period of years. It's not uncommon, for instance, for divorced parents who share the custody of children with ex-spouses to find that their conception of proper care progressively and seriously diverges from their former partner's as time goes on—even if they have known their spouses intimately for years, and reared the children with them for long periods. And, it seems unlikely that the people who conceived a child could get to know an adoptive parent as intimately as they know each other.

This doesn't mean that adoption is always wrong. It may well be the best option available for a child. When a pregnant woman (or, more often, a teenage child) decides she is unable to care for a baby and either chooses not to have an abortion, or, because of her beliefs or social constraints, finds that abortion is not an option, she may bear the baby and then give it up. She is doing what she can to see to it that the baby's needs are met, and this is praiseworthy. Sara Ruddick tells the story of a woman of her acquaintance who gave her baby up for adoption, not because she was *unable* to care for it, but because she figured that the child would have a better life elsewhere than the one she could provide.[7] Ruddick points out that this too is a gesture of care, and one that ought to be practiced more often. We regard it as more problematic, for the reason discussed above: if family members aren't interchangeable, the parents owe the child not the best available goods, but themselves. The child holds a claim of care, heritage, and place within the family against both mother and father, and it is too young to release them. All the same, we imagine that Ruddick's acquaintance found herself somewhere inside that gray area where the degree of hardship involved in honoring the child's claims might spur some to adopt and others to rear. Here, as in more clearcut cases of ordinary adoption, we have a response to an already-existing pregnancy that is somehow troublesome. Something has gone wrong. Some kind of calamity exists that prevents the parents from adequately supplying to the child what they owe her of their own persons.

If this analysis is close to accurate, then we can begin to see how certain reproductive technologies, notwithstanding their good intentions, threaten to further distort already undervalued and not-well-understood features of the parent-child relationship.

"Bob" the Sperm Vendor

The earliest form of assisted reproduction wasn't so very medical, although it now has high-tech medical features. Human pregnancy by artificial insemination dates to 1799, and by the 1890s there were instances of artificial insemination by a donor (other than a husband). Today it might be more accurate to call it artificial insemination by vendor, as the men involved are paid to provide the necessary sperm.

"Bob," an anonymous sperm vendor living near Philadelphia, sells his sperm to a bank as often as once a month. The going rate depends on the quantity of semen obtained, but is generally between fifty and one hundred dollars per ejaculation. Often the vendors are medical students recruited by sperm banks near or within the hospitals where they train; others, like "Bob," are simply young men from various walks of life who are willing to earn a little extra pocket money.

"Bob" sells his sperm to a private sperm bank in downtown

Philadelphia.[8] Most banks were housed in universities until the 1970s, when vasectomies became popular; then private banks were established to freeze and store sperm before the operation. Currently there are about a dozen large commercial sperm banks and at least fifteen smaller ones in the United States, along with any number of sperm storage facilities in physician's offices and teaching hospitals.[9]

To increase the likelihood of a successful pregnancy, frozen sperm is thawed and washed to separate it from other components of the semen, such as prostaglandins, antibodies, and microorganisms. The semen is then diluted with albumin or serum and centrifuged at low speed to separate out the sperm. The concentrated sperm are resuspended, then inserted with a syringe into a woman's cervical canal. In this way the procedure has become medicalized, but it is perfectly possible to get pregnant by artificial insemination without any medical help at all.

It is not, however, prudent to do so. In 1988 the American Fertility Society issued guidelines recommending that all use of fresh sperm be discontinued; the American College of Obstetricians and Gynecologists has endorsed these guidelines. The reason is that fresh sperm might be infected by HIV, the virus associated with AIDS, or with other microorganisms that don't belong inside the uterus. As HIV can't be detected until the infected person has had time to build up antibodies—a process that can take anywhere from three to six months—the sperm should be frozen for six months. At that time the donor would be tested, and if the test is positive, the frozen sperm discarded.

Because physicians perform the procedure (and because they supervise the banks where the frozen sperm is housed), artificial insemination must be thought of as a medical treatment. How, through the use of this procedure, does medicine distort what families can and should be? It deliberately severs the genetic strand of fatherhood from the nurturing and identity-forging strands, thereby perpetuating an ancient pattern in our culture of permitting men to impregnate women and then walk away. While such men have traditionally received some (rather mild) social censure—often accompanied by winks and jests—it is only very recently that the law and other social institutions have begun to reflect our understanding of how serious and widespread the problem of paternal abandonment is. Even if the parties consent to it and precautions are taken to employ only safe sperm, awarding this pattern a medical stamp of approval sends a very clear message to both men and women about the nature of their obligations to children they conceive.

Contract Pregnancy

A second medicalized approach to infertility also cuts the strands of parenthood apart. In contract pregnancy, a woman is hired to bear a child, usually for a couple who can't (or can't readily) have a child themselves. This woman is generally called a surrogate mother, but as it isn't very clear just who is standing surrogate for whom, it is probably better to drop the term and identify the woman within whose womb the fetus grows as the birthgiver. Finding a name for the woman, if any, to whom the baby is to be turned over at birth is less easy. She is usually the contracting father's wife, but it isn't useful to call her the contracting mother since the birthgiver too is a contracting mother, and besides, it is usually the father and not his wife who makes the contract with the birthgiver. So we will call her the social mother.

Of the two kinds of contract pregnancy, the vast majority involve the birthgiver's own egg and the contracting father's sperm, united through artificial insemination. No one keeps formal count of the number of these "traditional" contract pregnancies, but there have been somewhere upward of four thousand of them in the United States since the late 1970s.[10] The other kind, often called "gestational" contract pregnancy, has produced far fewer babies—perhaps eighty or so—because it involves hyperstimulation of the social mother's ovaries, retrieval of her eggs by means of an ultrasound-guided instrument passed through her vagina, fertilization of the eggs with her husband's sperm in a lab dish, and transfer of the resulting embryos to the birthgiver's uterus.

The cost to the couple for having a baby by contract is thirty to forty thousand dollars. About fifteen thousand of this is paid to the broker who arranges for the birth; there are at least twenty-nine contract pregnancy brokerages operating in the United States today. The birthgiver receives about ten to fifteen thousand for her services, and an additional ten thousand dollars or so goes to the birthgiver's medical, legal, insurance, and travel costs.[11] If the pregnancy is of the purely gestational variety, an extra ten to twelve thousand dollars will be spent on each attempt at in vitro fertilization, and because the success rate for IVF is low—the American

Fertility Society's 1990 figures put it at sixteen percent, although this varies from clinic to clinic—several attempts may be necessary. [12]

To date, five states—Arizona, Kentucky, Michigan, Utah, and Washington—have made it a crime to enter commercial pregnancy arrangements, and the contracts are unenforceable in another thirteen states (Arkansas, Florida, Indiana, Louisiana, Nebraska, Nevada, New Hampshire, New Jersey, New York, North Dakota, Oklahoma, Oregon, and Virginia). In some of these states the legal objection is to the exchange of money, which smacks of baby selling or prostitution, but in other states it is to the fate of the children should the contracts go awry; if an infant born sick or disabled is unwanted by the intended parents and the birthgiver as well, the child becomes a ward of the state. [13]

We too are worried about the fate of the children: here, as with artificial insemination by vendor, a situation is deliberately engineered that strips those responsible for the child's needs of the power to meet them. It isn't much like giving a child up for adoption, where a problem has already occurred that prevents those responsible for the child from rearing it themselves. Purposely creating the problem through a planned exchange is more like *disowning* the child—and that would seem to be a pretty clear instance of bad faith, whether or not money changes hands. As Janice Raymond has warned, even when a pregnancy is undertaken for the most altruistic of reasons—to provide a child for a close friend or a family member, for instance—subtle or blatant pressure might be exerted on the birthgiver to "be nice," to "give of herself," so that what looks like an act of altruism is really the product of coercion. Indeed, as Raymond points out, self-sacrifice for the good of others is so much a part of a patriarchal society's conception of what it is to be a woman that the widespread tendency to decry commercial surrogacy while celebrating altruistic surrogacy should be regarded with extreme suspicion. [14]

Too Many Parents and Not Enough

Putting more people into the reproductive chain of events produces subtle as well as obvious problems for artificial insemination by vendor and contract pregnancy. The obvious problem has already been discussed: directly causing a child to exist incurs responsibilities to the child that the causal agents have no intention of fulfilling. The subtle problem is that, while in contract pregnancy we think of the resulting child as having two mothers, in artificial insemination the sperm vendor is not commonly thought of as the child's father at all. So, in cases of contract pregnancy, if there is a dispute it's likely to be over who is the "real" mother, whereas in cases of artificial insemination, instead of having one father too many we sometimes end up with none.

Contract pregnancy and artificial insemination can avoid the charge of irresponsibility if arrangements are made to include the extra parent in the child's life in an ongoing and intimate way. Two gay men, for instance, could through contract pregnancy have a child who is genetically linked to one partner, so long as the mother of the child remained a visible and important part of the family. Such an arrangement would certainly be unusual, but it's difficult to see how a child could be harmed by stable relationships with a number of loving adults. The problem, of course, is that the couple might not welcome the intrusion of the third adult into their household; they might well see this as an intolerable invasion of their privacy. But while familial integrity is just as desirable in gay families as in straight ones, this doesn't mean that gay couples should model their households directly along the lines of heterosexual nuclear families. Creative and flexible alternatives have to be constructed. For example, the contract pregnancy might be undertaken on the understanding that the birthgiver is willing and able to visit the child on a regular basis in a noncustodial capacity, and that the custodial parents are willing to do all they can to encourage and cooperate with this arrangement.

For some lesbian parents a visible fatherly presence might be a workable solution to the problem of child rearing, but radical-separatist lesbians wouldn't find it acceptable, as their separatism is motivated by the belief that men reared in a patriarchal society are so damaged that they can't be trusted around women and children; they inflict too much harm. For women who believe this, it would be important to rear both their girl-children and their boy-children apart from men. Yet they too would be engineering a situation in which they produce children the fathers do not intend to rear. When they do this, are they acting in bad faith? Arguably, no. For these women, a tragedy of the sort that prompts adoption already exists; the evils inherent in the relationship between the sexes can't be undone in a generation. In this regard they are, like the woman who gives up her child for adoption because she can't rear him, doing the best they can under conditions of adversity.

Genetic Ties That Bind

Artificial insemination by vendor and contract pregnancy, the very infrequent practices of egg vending (at a going rate of two thousand dollars) or embryo donation, and even the less eye-catching reproductive technologies all have significant impact on society, not just because of the way they distort our understanding of the responsibilities of parenthood, but because of their strongly *genetic* orientation. The genes that are passed from generation to generation bear an enormous social significance. We think of them as the legacy we receive from our ancestors, as the fundamental source of our identity, as the link that binds us to our "real" parents. Both romantically and cynically, medicine alters these meanings.

THE CASE OF "BABY M"

At the same time as the genetic tie is thought to be precious, its moral significance under contract pregnancy is denied. In "traditional" contract pregnancy, the contracting father goes to a lot of trouble and expense to preserve his genetic link to his child, but the genetic link of the birthgiver he hires is played down, even though she contributes just as many genes as he does. We can see this clearly in the New Jersey case of "Baby M," where Mary Beth Whitehead, hired in 1985 to bear a child for William and Elizabeth Stern, refused to turn the baby over to the Sterns at birth and fled with her to Florida. The New Jersey trial court ruled that "surrogacy" contracts are enforceable and awarded sole custody of the baby to Mr. Stern, also granting Ms. Stern an order of adoption. When Ms. Whitehead appealed, the New Jersey Supreme Court ruled on 3 February 1988 that the contract was contrary to state statutes governing adoption and therefore not enforceable, but that it was in the child's best interests to be reared by her father; Ms. Whitehead was granted visitation rights. Because in most contested cases of contract pregnancy the father will be more affluent than the birthgiver and just as eager to rear the child, the courts are likely to find that the child is better off living with the father. The net effect is to privilege his biological connection to the child over the birthgiver's.

ANNA JOHNSON, INCUBATOR

In gestational contract pregnancy, the fact that the birthgiver has no genetic connection to the child has sometimes made all the difference. Crispina Calvert, unable to bear a child because she had had a hysterectomy, was nonetheless able to produce an egg that was fertilized in vitro with her husband Mark's sperm. The Calverts hired Anna Johnson, a black single mother with a three-year-old daughter, to gestate the embryo and turn over the resulting child to them for the standard fee of ten thousand dollars. Near the end of her pregnancy, Ms. Johnson asked the court to declare her the child's mother and sued for custody. After a hearing, Judge Richard N. Parslow, Jr., found that Anna Johnson had no parental rights. "She and the child are genetic hereditary strangers," the judge observed. "Anna's relationship to the child is analogous to that of a foster parent providing care, protection, and nurture during the period of time that the natural mother, Crispina Calvert, was unable to care for the child."[15]

The Court of Appeal agreed, finding it unnecessary to decide the two questions that had been raised in the "Baby M" case: whether the contract was enforceable and whether any particular custody arrangement was in the child's best interests. Instead, the appellate court focused exclusively on the question of which of the two women was the child's "natural" mother. The court decided that a blood test—a genetic test—should determine maternity, just as it could determine paternity under California law. It was rational to use genes instead of gestation to determine parenthood, said the court, because

> the whole process of human development "is set in motion by the genes." There is not a single organic system of the human body not influenced by an individual's underlying genetic makeup. Genes determine the way physiological components of the human body, such as the heart, liver, or blood vessels operate. Also, according to the expert testimony received at trial, it is now thought that genes influence tastes, preferences, personality styles, manners of speech and mannerisms.[16]

It's really quite remarkable to see how the genetic tie is valorized here, considering how firmly (and cynically) we shut our eyes to it in cases of anonymous artificial insemination. What would Bob the Sperm Vendor think of the appellate court's argument in the *Calvert* decision?

Freezing Future Generations

To impregnate Anna Johnson, the Calverts used in vitro fertilization, a technique that generally involves producing more fertilized eggs than will be needed. Here's how it works: a woman's ovaries are stimulated by fertility drugs to produce several ripe eggs at once. These are removed from the ovaries by ultrasonic transvaginal oocyte retrieval—a method that supersedes earlier retrieval systems requiring small incisions into the woman's abdomen. The eggs are then placed in a petrie dish, where they are united with sperm that has been washed, concentrated, and resuspended. Sperm and eggs are incubated for twelve to eighteen hours so that fertilization can occur, and then, after an additional forty-eight to seventy-two hours, preembryos will have formed. They are called preembryos until the appearance (fourteen days after fertilization) of the embryonic axis, or primitive streak, which initiates the development of the nervous system and marks the future symmetry of the human body.

At the four- to sixteen-cell stage, some of the preembryos will be put into a catheter that is threaded through the cervix and into the uterus—usually the uterus of the woman whose eggs were used, although in the Calvert-Johnson case they went into the hired birthgiver's uterus. But not all the preembryos will be used. And the question then becomes what to do with the ones that are left over.

Does one save them or throw them away? Often they are discarded, in which case it would seem the genetic material they contain doesn't matter very much after all. Paradoxically, these same embryos can be laden with enormous significance for both good and ill, should the parties involved decide to save them.

Because IVF doesn't work most of the time, and because getting the eggs out of a woman's body in the first place is difficult even with the new retrieval technologies, there is an incentive to freeze at least some unused preembryos for future attempts at IVF in case the present attempt proves a failure. This is so even though the success rate with frozen preembryos is only about half of what it is for fresh.[17]

How many frozen preembryos are currently sitting in storage? It's impossible to say, but estimates run to the tens of thousands. In 1990 alone, 129 clinics in the U.S. reported freezing 23,865 embryos. In that same year more than 290 babies were born from frozen preembryos.[18]

These numbers indicate that the freezing of human embryos is more than a scientific curiosity. "Steadily," the lawyer Ellen Moskowitz notes, "the technology is spreading. This lends an urgency to the moral and legal questions the technology raises."[19]

IS MR. DAVIS ALREADY A FATHER?

The legal question of what to do with frozen embryos was asked and answered most dramatically in Tennessee, in a case that at one point produced the strangest judicial decision for joint custody in the annals of American law. Mary Sue and Junior Davis badly wanted children, but their attempts to have them through intercourse led to five dangerous ectopic pregnancies. They tried to adopt a child, but at the last moment the child's birth mother changed her mind. They came to believe that IVF was their only hope.

Mary Sue went through seven cycles of IVF between 1985 and 1988, freezing only the embryos that resulted from the last cycle. Each time the eggs were retrieved, not by the new ultrasound-guided technique, but by the older, more invasive method of laparoscopic surgery. Neither Mary Sue nor her husband gave any thought to what should be done with the frozen embryos in the event the marriage came to an end or both partners died, nor did the clinic raise the question. Before the embryos were thawed and implanted, Junior Davis sued for divorce. He and Mary Sue agreed on all the terms of the divorce except the disposition of the embryos, which Mary Sue wanted to have implanted but Junior did not. They turned to the courts to settle the dispute.

The Tennessee trial court, terming the embryos "in vitro children," decided the embryos' interests would best be served by implantation, and awarded "custody" to Mary Sue to pursue this end. Junior appealed. By the time the Court of Appeals of Tennessee decided the case, Mary Sue and Junior were both remarried, and Mary Sue no longer wanted to bring the embryos to term herself. She did, however, want to donate them to a childless couple. The appeals court, rejecting the notion that embryos were "children" and focusing instead on the adults' interests, ruled that either party contributing a gamete to an embryo had veto power over implantation. The court awarded joint custody of the embryos to both Junior and Mary Sue. Mary Sue appealed.

The Tennessee Supreme Court rejected the appeals court's "veto" ruling that gave more weight to avoiding procreation than to pursuing procreation. First, the court concluded that if the Davises had made an agreement about the disposition of the embryos, the agreement would have been a binding contract, enforceable by the Tennessee courts. But because there was no such agreement, the court invoked the notion of a balancing test to determine what result would impose the least personal suffering and hardship on the disputants. Deciding that Mary Sue's interest in donating the embryos was not as significant as Junior's interest in avoiding paternity, the court ruled in favor of Junior. In 1993 the United States Supreme Court declined to hear the case, but that was not the end of the litigation: the fertility clinic, which has a policy against directly destroying frozen embryos, asked the Tennessee trial court to order the transfer of the embryos to another clinic for disposal. According to sources close to the case who have asked to remain anonymous, the embryos finally ended up in Junior Davis's keeping, and in spring of 1993 he took them to a river and ceremoniously released them into the water.

It seems to us that the Tennessee courts have taken a stance that might be called false gender neutrality—denying that gender is relevant when in fact it is. Ordinarily, we don't regard men and women on an equal footing with respect to fertilized eggs; once the man has contributed his sperm, he's made his decision (in effect) to be a father. Whether he actually turns out to be a parent is a matter of fate and the decision of the pregnant woman, who (for reasons we argued earlier), must retain the right to stop the pregnancy. The Tennessee courts were likely confused by the fact that Mary Sue was not harboring the embryos in her body; such harboring is the clearest source of the different moral authority of women and men concerning pregnancy. What the courts overlooked, though, was the gender difference apparent in how those embryos made their way to the freezer. The nature of Junior's task in contributing gametes was straightforward, possibly even pleasant: male bodies are designed to discharge gametes rather easily. Women's bodies, on the other hand, are built so as to house gametes rather than ejaculate them. Getting eggs into a petrie dish meant ingesting potentially carcinogenic chemicals and undergoing repeated operations for Mary Sue, and even with the newer retrieval techniques, a woman endures procedures that are so invasive that they'd constitute a serious violation of her person if she hadn't consented to them. Such consent, it should be noted, is predicated on certain understandings—crucially, that the harvested eggs are to be used for the purpose of bringing a child into the world. It's not enough for the male partner to have "changed his mind."

To see this, consider the following analogy. Suppose a great classical violinist is losing his manual dexterity, and can only hope to continue to give concert performances if he submits to a painful, somewhat risky operation on both hands. As it happens, there is only one surgeon who can perform this procedure, and, being a fan of classical music she agrees to do it. The surgeon's protocol is to do just one hand at a time, allowing the first to heal before the second operation is attempted. However, after the first operation, she becomes converted to atonal music, and finds that she has nothing but contempt for the classical repertoire. She therefore refuses to complete the operation.

That the surgeon is acting unethically here is not likely to be questioned; she's violating a contract and is liable to be sued. But, on reflection, it seems clear that this isn't just a civil matter for which money damages are appropriate compensation. The surgeon's agreement to do *both* halves of the operation was the basis of her patient's consent to the surgery in the first place. In refusing to operate on the second hand, the surgeon has in effect changed the meaning of the first operation. It's no longer the initial step in a process that will give the violinist back his career. Instead, it's a painful and invasive procedure that's no longer a part of what the patient consented to, and that makes it a form of assault. So is the bodily invasion required for in vitro fertilization if the partner changes his mind in midstream about wanting a child.

The surgeon's shift in musical allegiance and Mr. Davis's shift in his desire to father children with Ms. Davis both illustrate an interesting moral phenomenon we have marked earlier: in morality, the future can, as it were, alter the past. Just as an adult child's rejection of his parents can make their earlier relationship instrumental, so too can a unilateral change of purpose transform what was a shared, cooperative relationship into a relationship of exploitation.

In the case of the dispute between Junior and Mary Sue, Mary Sue has now changed her mind as well. She no longer wants to bring these embryos to term herself, but rather to allow other women to do so. Does her change of mind allow Junior the freedom to change his own?

Disputes and hard questions like these arise because advances in biomedical technology produce categories of family members society has never had to deal with before. A preembryo is not a child, but it's more like a child than, say, a kidney is.[20] A woman who carries another couple's embryo to term is sort of like a wet-nurse, but she is also a birthgiver and so a mother. As a result of our categorical confusions, law and society are hard put to figure out when to hold people responsible for their genetic ties. In the case of the Calverts the responsibility is judged to be self-evident. But not in the case of Bob the Sperm Vendor; not in the case of postmenopausal women who can now, thanks to egg donation and IVF, experience pregnancy and give birth to children who are not genetically related to them; not in the case of Junior Davis.

The examples we've canvassed reveal striking inconsistencies in the way our society construes the importance of genetic connection. The quick explanation of these inconsistencies is that society has left the construction of this meaning up to the individual. It's a question of private choice. Each of us can decide for ourselves how important the genetic tie is: if it's very important to both partners in a heterosexual relationship, they'll arrange for a gestational contract pregnancy; if it's important only to the father (or to both members of the gay couple), the partners will choose "traditional" contract pregnancy; if it isn't important at all, the prospective parents (or single parent) will adopt.

The trouble with leaving the individual to decide what the genetic link should mean is that meaning doesn't often remain private. A public understanding of the importance of our genes is likely to emerge from these private decisions—but it will not have been arrived at through public discussion and consensus. Moreover, because the private decisions take place in a medical context, they are biased toward bodily interventions (which is what makes them medical, after all) and hence the genetic tie is easily manipulated. IVF becomes a means of achieving a genetic tie despite the fact that the fallopian tubes are blocked or nonexistent. Contract pregnancies are a bid to keep at least one genetic line open, as is artificial insemination by vendor—where, in addition, the woman to be inseminated is presented with a genetic "menu" (blond hair, height 6'2", and other such characteristics of the various vendors) to help her select the most desirable sperm. Rather than allowing this scientific and technological bias to determine, by accident, what such concepts as "mother," "father," "parenthood," and "family" are to mean in American society, we would do well to think these questions through in a public dialogue.

Advances in biomedical technology have given peoples' genetic ties to their offspring a new visibility even in cases where subfertility is not at issue. Routine genetic screening also subtly alters our understanding of what it means to form a family.

ONE DOWN SYNDROME TOO MANY

We ran into her in San Francisco, in one of those coincidences that leaves people murmuring about how small a world it is. We were walking up Nob Hill in the early spring sunshine on the way back to our hotel when we caught sight of Corinne across the street. Although we still wrote to each other every two years or so, we hadn't seen her in ten, and we weren't quite sure it was she until she hailed us. In the hour before she was due at the airport we sat at a sidewalk café and brought ourselves up to date.

She was in town on business, she said, and she still lived in Oregon with her husband and two children. We had met the oldest child when he was a newborn, but the toddler was news. "And how's your mother?" I asked. "Do you remember when we were about ten years old and your mother helped us build our treehouse?"

"It's still up in that tree. Mother's doing okay for a seventy-five-year-old lady. She's slowed down a lot, though."

"And Sarah Frances?" I remembered Sarah Frances as sunny, obstreperous, clamoring to be allowed to play with us though she was ten years older than we. Sarah Frances had Down syndrome.

"She died last year of kidney failure."

"Oh, Corinne. I'm sorry."

Corinne nodded. "But it was a relief, too. Mother had been worrying about what would happen when she got too old to take care of her by herself. I told her we'd take her, but Mother said it would be hard on the children."

"I always thought you were very good with Sarah Frances."

"She was sweet. Even so, it was a tough way to grow up. And now, in a funny, superstitious sort of way, I feel like I somehow caused her to die."

"What on earth—"

"Oh, I just mean I feel guilty. I never told you about it—it wasn't the kind of thing I could put in a letter—but I thought maybe I'd tell you both the next time I saw you, so I guess I will." She stopped talking and frowned at the geraniums separating our table from the sidewalk. The petals, a splash of scarlet in the sunlight, held their own against the fuschia suit of a woman walking by.

"When Adam was six I got pregnant again. We planned it—I'd just finished my MBA and Mike and I both thought that if we waited much longer Adam would feel like an only child all his life. I had amniocentesis, of course—I'd had it when I was carrying Adam too, because of Sarah Frances. Only this time the trisomy was present."

"The fetus had Down syndrome."

Corinne nodded again, her eyes still fixed on the red geraniums in their clean white boxes. "Mike was terrific about it, said of course we'd love the baby and take good care of her—it was a girl—but he knew he didn't really know what we were in for. Neither did I, since she might have been only mildly retarded, or maybe she'd be far worse off than Sarah Frances. You can't tell ahead of time. The awful thing was that I'd already started to make friends with the baby—you know how you do when you're pregnant?"

I did.

"Well, we went round and round on it for a week, with Mike saying he'd go along with whatever I thought best and me wishing it was Mike's decision so I wouldn't have to be responsible for it. But I finally decided I couldn't go through it all again. I loved Sarah Frances—really loved her, I mean—but she was a burden, too. I didn't want that for Adam. And I was watching Mother worry about what would happen if Sarah Frances outlived her, and thinking I'd have that worry too some day."

The sun was making small rainbow shimmers in Corinne's sleek dark hair. She turned her head and gave us a little grin. "I had the abortion. We were awfully sad about it, even though we thought we were doing the right thing. But when Amanda was born she was even more precious to us because of the other baby that didn't ever get to live. I've often wondered, though, just what I was saying about Sarah Frances when I had that abortion."

If contract pregnancy and artificial insemination invite us to pick among various individual meanings for reproductive events, a similar pick-and-choose model is introduced by genetic screening. With amniocentesis and newer, more sophisticated techniques for detecting genetic conditions, there is a medical assumption that parents ought to decide which babies they want to bring into the world. *Family matters are stuck with each other* no longer.

This is of course not necessarily a bad thing. Corinne's decision not to hold her family hostage to the same ill fortune that had been her own lot in childhood is surely one we can sympathize with. Down syndrome and certain other genetic diseases cannot be cured, but genetic screening allows us to stop the pregnancies that produce them—arguably a better alternative than watching a child with, say, Tay-Sachs disease die slowly and painfully.

At the same time, there is something both romantic and cynical about insisting on the primacy of one's freedom to choose or reject intimates. It is romantic because it places a high premium on personal liberty, on the value of entering into relationships of one's own free will. And it is cynical because it applies notions of quality control to human beings, in a kind of pessimistic shrewdness that establishes a means of escape from potential relationships that don't come up to standard. When families use medicine as a means to that freedom, they romanticize medicine as well. There can be a cost to this. Medical mechanisms that help families exercise great freedom in choosing who will enter the next generation can endanger something that is central to the ethos of families: the value of accepting people as they are, of making the best of things within the intimate relationships one has not chosen.

Moreover, when genetic screening becomes a routine method of eliminating defective fetuses, choice itself can become a burden. As Barbara Katz Rothman puts it:

> The potential for pregnancy loss, through abortion, is built right into amniocentesis. Terminating a wanted pregnancy at twenty weeks is a profoundly wrenching, painful experience. The potential for such a termination casts its shadow back over the entire first half of the pregnancy, creating the "tentative pregnancy." A woman's commitment to her pregnancy under the conditions imposed by amniocentesis can

only be tentative. She cannot ignore it, but neither can she wholeheart-edly embrace it. The pregnancy may not be leading to a baby, but to an abortion.

Women usually manage to keep the anxiety under control—we are strong—but there is a cost to that: the cost is in the developing relation-ship with the fetus, and the woman's developing sense of herself as the baby's mother.[21]

The pregnant woman's continual process of making friends with her fetus, an important mechanism for drawing new members into the family, is indeed distorted and interrupted by the long wait for the results of the amniocentesis to be known. But just as difficult, perhaps, is the burden imposed on the family by the opportunity to assess—and hence the necessity to assess—the quality of the "product" that might become a family member unless it is weighed and found wanting.

These reservations about genetic screening's impact on the family must, however, be put into their proper historical context. It wasn't so very long ago that American families experienced not merely tentative pregnancies, but tentative infancies. In the days before immunization and decent sanitation, many babies died—as they still do, in southern coun-tries—of dysentery, typhoid, diphtheria, and other lethal diseases. "If he lives," a sailor might write home on learning of the birth of a son, "name him John." We can only guess at the extent to which families held back some part of themselves on account of their infants' precarious hold on existence.

We owe twentieth-century medicine a considerable debt for its share in securing the safety of our own babies. And it's important to acknowl-edge that genetic screening is an invaluable tool for diminishing significantly what could otherwise be a catastrophe of serious propor-tions. All the same, widespread use of amniocentesis and other genetic screens does have a subtle yet durable impact on the way families perpet-uate themselves, and the way they relate to their newest members.

The work of the Human Genome Project and other federally sponsored research has already produced markers allowing doctors to identify, early in pregnancy, such diseases as Huntington chorea, adult onset polycystic kidney disease, and others that won't produce visible symptoms unless the fetus grows into an adult. With these disorders, a person might have a very good life for quite a long while before disease overtakes her. Is it right to stop a pregnancy simply because one foreknows what will happen to its issue in thirty or forty years? Such foreknowledge is of course only an illusion; none of us can know another's end. The world is riddled with perils—with car accidents, with drug addiction, with cancers that strike the young. In stopping the pregnancy merely because one knows of a specific hazard, when so many others are unknown, mightn't one tacitly be acting as if one must guarantee one's children a full and long life? One doesn't hurt the person that the fetus might have become by stopping the pregnancy, as the person then will never exist; however, one might damage the family as a whole if one acts as if parents have a duty to their potential and present children to shield them from many decades of harm.

Genetic Screening and Abortion

In addition to the genetic markers already discovered, others will likely be found for serious conditions such as schizophrenia and manic depressive disorder, as well as for less severe conditions such as obesity, freckling, myopia, behavioral problems, and learning disorders. As these lesser conditions become predictable, will families be tempted to get frivolously fussy about which pregnancies will be brought to term and which will not? And is there anything wrong with such fussiness?

Imagine two pregnancies. In the first, a woman who is using a drug for her migraine headaches is told she ought not to become pregnant while taking it, because the resulting child is likely to have a withered arm. If she discontinues the drug and waits two months, she is likely to bear a perfectly normal child. She considers this and decides she doesn't want to wait. She gets pregnant. The child has a withered arm.[22]

Her behavior seems selfish, doesn't it? With just a little patience and no real cost to herself she might have had a child with sound limbs. It wouldn't have been *this* child, but no necessity drove her to have this child. She just didn't want to wait, and so put a little extra misery into the world that could easily have been avoided.

Compare her to another woman, newly pregnant at some point in the near future when a routine genetic screen on the seventh day of pregnancy is capable of indicating that the preembryo she carries will become a seriously overweight person. The gene for obesity, she is told, is recessive, so if she aborts this fetus and tries again, she very likely will have a child who is not obese. She decides to continue the pregnancy. Yet with just a little patience and no real cost to herself she might have had a child of normal proportions. She just didn't want to wait, and so put a little extra misery into the world that could easily have been avoided.

The cases are different, of course. About the first case one might say that there is no generally recognized duty to begin any one particular life, although (in the second case) there might be a duty not to stop a life once it has begun. We think there probably is such a duty, even if it is far from absolute, and even it must always be assessed within the context of existing social structures (where women haven't necessarily had a great deal to say about when they would become pregnant or who would provide the care once the child was born). The duty not to stop a pregnancy is grounded in the idea that if a fetus is allowed to develop, it becomes a morally considerable child, with an interest in living its life and with a wide range of valuable experiences in its future.[23]

In our two comparison cases, the question isn't one of perpetuating a systemic injustice against women: the problem with the pregnancy isn't, for example, that the future child's father refuses to assume his responsibilities care and so forces the mother to postpone other life-projects as she bears the full burden of nurturing the child. Nor, we will assume, is she so dependent on the father that intercourse and consequent pregnancy is a necessary means of assuring her economic or emotional well-being. Bracketing those concerns for a moment, then, we can return to the cases and ask what an ethics of the family might have to say about them.

One consequence of framing the problem this way is to shift the focus from the individual to the collective. Instead of puzzling over what is in the mother's best interests, or whether one can speak at all of the interests of a person who does not yet exist, we can set these pregnancies in their familial context, where they function to renew and extend the family.

Is there a precedent within families for screening prospective candidates for membership? Indeed there is, as anyone who has ever brought a suitor home to meet the folks can tell you. Premarital screening is the family's way of protecting itself, the idea being to avert lasting harm if the suitor should prove to be a person of bad character or should his disability or illness threaten to drain the family's resources. The screening

Corinne underwent was analogous to this. Very different is the sort of screening that rejects a prospective family member on the basis of obesity or a withered arm.

When families allow relatively trivial physical criteria of this kind to determine eligibility for membership, they endanger one of their most important moral features: the feature of loving acceptance. While praiseworthy in any individual who happens to possess it, loving acceptance is crucial for families, because it is the basis for the trust that holds them together. We wrote in Chapter Two of the family's ability to impart to its members a sense of belonging, and how this is crucial for forming and maintaining the self. If this sense is undermined by a fear that family membership is contingent on physical completeness—if illness, frailty, or disability means that home is no longer "the place where, when you have to go there, / They have to take you in"—then the family has stopped being a family and become something more like a country club.[24] Having lost sight of the idea that *Family members are stuck with each other* the family adopts an ethos in which relationships are based on contract and consent. Advances in genetic screening are unwitting forces pushing the family in this direction.

When the Fetus Joins the Family

Because fetuses are now much more visible than they used to be, thanks not only to amniocentesis but to endoscopy, ultrasound, alpha-fetoprotein assays, and the new fetal surgeries, there's some point to asking at what point the fetus joins the family. Is fetal surgery, for example, obligatory when medically indicated even though the fetus can only be reached by major incisions into the mother's body? What other sorts of familial sacrifices must be made on the fetus's behalf? The new fetal visibility has permitted a new level of social intrusion into the family's affairs. What social messages do pregnant women receive when they are confronted by large notices in bars exhorting them to look after the health of their unborn children? What social messages are conveyed by criminal prosecution of women who refuse delivery by cesarean section when birth is complicated by placenta previa?

In Oakland County, California, on 23 April 1993, the chief executive officer of the county hospital system announced that Trisha Marshall, killed by a bullet to the head while in her seventeenth week of pregnancy, would be kept on life-support at Highland General Hospital as long as there was any hope that her fetus could be brought to term. It was. A baby boy was delivered by cesarean section on 3 August, 105 days after his mother was declared brain dead. Leaving to one side the major consideration that this technology, when it succeeds at all, is likely to produce a severely low-birthweight baby with many physical problems, what social message does the decision to continue the pregnancy convey about a mother's duties even after death? Would the family be censured if they sought to honor the dead by requesting Ms. Marshall's body for burial? If life-support under these circumstances becomes routine, we will have yet another instance of biomedical technology putting pressure on family members to make new and strange sacrifices for each other. The window medicine has opened into women's wombs intensifies a romantic view of motherhood.[25]

Medicine's view of the meaning of reproduction—a view that families are increasingly coming to share—has on the whole not been good for families. Its selective exaggeration at one moment and denial at the next of the importance of genetic ties makes it easy to lose sight of what families are like and why they matter. When we endow the brute physical genetic link with intense significance, we are groping clumsily for a deep, rich, and full connection to past and future generations. But in that groping we have taken one element of reproduction and enshrined it as the crucial one. From a social rather than a biological perspective, the gene is, after all, only a shoddy proxy for a clear and complete connection to the family's ongoing story—a connection that families provide for in many other ways. Marriage, for example, augments the existing history rather than replicating it genetically; so might living under the same roof for a long period of time, as stepsiblings sometimes do. Adoption and the long intimate friendships that make us think of a person as a metaphoric aunt, brother, or grandfather—are all ancient mechanisms by which the family pulls new people into its orbit. The friction between families and medicine might be relieved to some degree if, rather than relying so heavily on genetic ties, families could remember to look to some of their other traditional mechanisms for extending and preserving themselves.

Chapter Seven

With Medicine and Justice for All

ON A MORNING RIDE INTO NEW YORK ON THE METRO NORTH LINE, A commuter's heart-lifting view of the Hudson River and the Palisade hills soon gives way to a very different scene. As Grand Central Station approaches, the train slides by a new hospital set squarely in the middle of a very depressed and very depressing part of town. The hospital has an ICU gleaming with up-to-the-minute technology, and is staffed by doctors and administrators whose Jaguars, Volvos, and Saabs line the parking lot. A few minutes later, the train passes a graffiti-splashed school without windows, where nothing is new except the metal detectors, and to which no one drives fancy cars. And in between are countless apartments, many housing families who have almost no access to health care at all.

The moral view from the commuter's seat reveals striking imbalances in the way we distribute our social resources. Health care is a big winner; education is doing much less well. The view from within families is no better proportioned. Not only are some families far poorer than others, but within households the labor of day-to-day living tends to fall disproportionately heavily on its adult women, while other burdens and benefits are also skewed, slighting in some families the old, in some the young, and in some particular individuals for what seem completely idiosyncratic reasons.

All these contrasts are both pronounced and quite familiar, but they may not seem to be importantly related. Instances of social injustice bear a surface resemblance to beads on a string: the string that connects them is the injustice itself, but the beads don't seem to have anything else in common—there appears to be no significant connection between, say, unfairness in families and unfairness in health care. A commuter into New York sees a representative sample of our worst social problems every day— poverty, homelessness, urban decay, economic stagnation, environmental degradation. Why should she think that issues of equitable access to health care have anything in common with issues of justice in the way we structure family life?

Surprisingly enough, there *are* deep and interesting connections between the two, with implications for both our theoretical and practical understanding of justice in the institutions of health care and the family. As a matter of theory, the ideas of justice that have been a part of our intellectual heritage will have to be recast pretty thoroughly if we're to get a clear sense of what justice within families or medicine might become, because both institutions have similar—and similarly misunderstood— ways of structuring the personal relationships at their cores. As a matter of practice, we need to get a better understanding of how the patterns of injustice in medicine and families actually feed off each other. The expectations that medicine entertains about families and that families entertain about medicine are part of a host of forces that seem to be sinking both institutions deeper into the mire. Family members tend to believe that medicine can and will do "everything" for their sick loved ones, thus demanding treatment that contributes to the fiscal crisis in health care, while medicine looks to families to take over more of the work of care that has traditionally gone on in medical settings, thus deepening the injustices in the distribution of caring labor that are already endemic to families.

The Problem of Justice Comes to the Fore
There are signs that America may be starting to emerge from a long, stubborn period of corporate denial about the glaring problems of justice

facing the institutions of family and medicine. President Clinton's election made health care reform almost an obsession; the phenomenon of tens of millions of under- and uninsured Americans excluded from access to decent health care, combined with the problem of steep rises in an already immense health care budget, finally caught the attention of the public and lawmakers alike. There's something eye-catchingly unjust in spending fifteen percent of the GNP on health care while the same percentage of our citizens have no insured entry into the system. At the same time, people seem increasingly disturbed by at least the more egregious instances of familial injustice: those for example, of fathers who run away from their parental responsibilities.[1]

We're seeing some interesting developments: corporate leaders are now calling for a medical system which only a few short years before they would have condemned as "socialist." Slowly but steadily, company policies are recognizing that family life has to continue despite the fact that fewer and fewer men have a wife at home to keep house (women, of course, never had wives at all, unless you count those whose husbands were rich enough to afford servants). But although we are beginning to acknowledge that injustice in both families and medicine can no longer be ignored, the specific patterns by which this injustice plays itself out in the two systems isn't generally seen to raise theoretical problems, nor has much attention been paid to how practical and theoretical patterns complicate and reinforce each other. Here's an illustration of how such reinforcement works.

ANOTHER WOMAN IN THE MIDDLE

The digital clock on the microwave flashed to 12:00 and Wednesday tumbled into Thursday as Jamie rather numbly stirred the cocoa and sugar together in the pan, preparing the ritual hot chocolate which served as her tranquilizer every night. Tom's father, newly home from the hospital, was still recovering from his heart attack and had been having a bad evening; he had been fratchety and demanding. Tom's son was going through the breakup of yet another intense relationship and had needed a good deal of comforting himself. And Tom? Well, he had been snoring for about an hour now. Tom's wife, Jamie reflected, was getting pretty tired of the whole thing, particularly with three classes' worth of student papers left ungraded.

DR. SCHLIERMACHER'S CHOICE

Tom's father's cardiologist, Dr. Schliermacher, is well known for his strong commitment to his patients and sensitivity to their families. One mark of this commitment is that his drug of choice for patients experiencing a heart attack is tissue plasminogen activator, or t-PA. This genetically engineered agent is administered as soon as the patient reaches the emergency room, to destroy the blood clot that's preventing oxygen from reaching the heart muscle. If the clot can be dissolved so blood can flow through the artery, the damage to the heart muscle will be much less severe. The drug costs twenty-four hundred dollars per dose, compared to four hundred dollars for a dose of streptokinase, another drug that also dissolves blood clots. Studies of their relative benefit have been contradictory, and it's probably fair to say the overall evidence hasn't demonstrated any unambiguous advantages to the use of t-PA, but it's certainly no worse than streptokinase and probably marginally better. In a recent study, sixty-three out of one thousand patients given t-PA died within thirty days of their heart attacks, compared to seventy-three out of one thousand patients given streptokinase. T-PA does carry a 1.3 percent chance of causing a debilitating stroke, but then, streptokinase produces a severe allergic reaction in 1.5 percent of patients. So, t-PA is perhaps slightly more effective. "A doctor does not make his decision based on price," says Dr. Schliermacher. "If we can say that t-PA is better, then we have to give it."[2]

Tom's dad got t-PA, because Tom's dad, like all the doctor's patients, is worth it. Occasionally, Dr. Schliermacher's colleagues press him a little about the extra cost, and he says that he would be willing to talk over the decision with the patient or the patient's family—he's the sort of doctor who's willing to talk about almost anything. But you have to get a thrombolytic agent into the patient fast—preferably within the first hour of the heart attack, so there's not much time for a prolonged conversation. Besides, it doesn't typically cost patients or their families any more to use t-PA, since the insurance company picks up the tab. And so, Dr. Schliermacher assumes, they aren't likely to reason about this issue in any way other than he does. In making this assumption, he is certainly right, as least as far as Jamie, Tom, and Tom's father are concerned.

These snippets of a story hint at both kinds of interconnection between the justice problems facing families and medicine to which we've already alluded. Jamie is tired and disgruntled at the end of a long and unusually taxing day—life can be tough in families—but she loves her father-in-law, her son, and her husband, they all love her, and their love is expressed everyday in many subtle, hard-to-measure ways. Tom's not much good at comforting the sick or the lovelorn, but he certainly keeps the car going, and is reasonably cheerful about chauffeuring the kids around; occasionally, it is his hand that stirs Jamie's nightly hot cocoa while she grabs a few delicious minutes of reading in bed. Is that atmosphere going to thrive if she starts insisting on an exacting standard of parity? She may hammer out a "comparable work" standard: so many minutes spent soothing a son versus so many oil changes. What will the family feel like if Tom has to fill out the kind of time-sheets at home that he grumbles over at work every week?

As for Dr. Schliermacher's use of t-PA rather than streptokinase, once again the question seems to be a matter of understanding what the philosopher F. H. Bradley called "our station and its duties." When something goes wrong with your heart, do you want a cardiologist or an accountant? Is Dr. Schliermacher a health policy analyst or a physician? For just whose interests is he supposed to be a faithful advocate—his patients', or their insurance companies'?

For both Jamie and Dr. Schliermacher, things seem to be as they ought. As a matter of fact, there are serious questions of justice hidden in each story. In Jamie's story, the hidden injustice is that caring for people—typically women's work—is unlike caring for a car. It costs the caregiver in countless, unnoticed ways. In Dr. Schliermacher's story, the hidden injustice is the effect on the health care system when neither the caregiver, the patient, nor the patient's family, pays any attention to the price of the treatment.

The fact that neither medicine nor families are especially good at embodying justice hardly distinguishes them from other institutions in our culture. Nor are their interrelations the only problems each faces in the struggle to be just. But these stories suggest that in our society it's not terribly clear that justice as a moral standard is even applicable to families or medicine. And, as we'll see presently, our society's uncertainty feeds into a pattern of expectation for both families and medicine in which each makes it harder for the other to do what's right.

Favoritism and Justice

Let's start with the question of whether justice is really an appropriate standard for the kind of intimate relationships we hope will flourish in families and between patients and physicians. You can't think very long about either families or medicine—or have read very far in this book, at any rate—without being struck by the special character of their moral commitments. As social institutions, families and medicine both are built on the idea of favoritism: our relatives, or our patients, have a call on our loyalty in ways that distinguish them from others who don't stand in such relationships with us. That's why we have trouble thinking about these institutions as the kinds of places where justice should prevail: justice doesn't play favorites.

There is, to be sure, a great deal of controversy about what justice demands of us. Some theorists see it as requiring that all property be held in common.[3] Others think justice leaves us free to step over starving children in the road, so long as we don't default on any of our contracts.[4] Despite this diversity, there is a widely accepted core to the concept that doesn't seem very hospitable to the idea of special loyalties. To be just, fundamentally, is to treat those things that are relevantly alike, alike, and to treat those things that are relevantly different, differently. Determining what is "relevantly alike" or "relevantly different" is precisely how a great deal of the practical and theoretical arguments about justice begin, but it is generally agreed that we can only determine what is or is not relevant if we start with the assumption that everyone deserves equal consideration, and that no one is privileged because of whom she might know, or to whom he might happen to be related.

Both the notion of just treatment and the notion of special loyalty are central to the way in which many of us make moral sense of our experience—including our experience of families and the health care system. But, on the face of it, these notions don't fit together very well. If we are to understand the moral relationship between families, medicine, and other parts of our life—indeed, if we want to avoid moral incoherence generally—we need to see the tension between impartialism and favoritism more clearly, and come up with thoughtful strategies to ease it. Only then can we understand how the reform of the health care system and the equally essential reform of the family are tasks that interpenetrate, and how the quest for justice in either sphere should be shaped by the quest for justice in the other.

THE KINDNESS OF STRANGERS

Richard Barrie walked along the beach with us, making a strenuous effort to keep the conversation light, until we reached the particular cove that was his favorite. We had gotten to know him well in a summer-vacation sort of way, as our little cottage sat closely behind his beachfront villa and our children had been good playmates over the years. Ordinarily we orbited in very different social circles—he owned a string of television stations and had large shares in several advertising agencies—but children, sand, and wet bathing suits are great levelers and on Lake Erie we met as equals.

There was a large, sun-splashed rock jutting out into the cove. Richard scrambled up onto it, still making small talk, while we climbed up beside him. I could almost reach the bramble of wild roses cascading down the face of the cliff. We all fell silent, looking out over the water, and it was some minutes before Richard spoke.

"You know, she's never complained. Oh, I guess that's not strictly true. Any five-year-old kid who's been through all the operations she's had to go through is going to complain a little here and there, but she's always been so damned sunny and good-natured about everything. Of course we've all petted her. Having four big brothers and sisters who treat her like a china doll should by rights have spoiled her rotten—I dunno why it didn't. And yet there's not one of us that can give Margaret the heart and lungs and liver and bowels she needs to keep alive. Wouldn't you think that out of such a large family there'd be a good match for a kidney, at least?"

"Has Pittsburgh agreed to do the transplants?"

"Yeah—as soon as we can find the donors. Multiple transplant candidates don't go on the regular waiting list, so as soon as the organs become available . . . But there's not much time." Richard's glance followed a gull's flight over the treetops and he swallowed hard.

"We've started a broadcast campaign. I've spent the last couple of days taping the appeal and we'll begin airing it tomorrow. It's worked before, for other kids. Last year there was that little girl in England. That was a six-organ transplant too, and the publicity worked—they got the organs."

Behind Richard's back we exchanged quick, worried looks. We remembered the case. That little girl, born like Margaret without a bowel, had gotten the organs and the transplantation center at the University of Pittsburgh had performed the operation, but the child died. Nobody so far had ever survived the procedure.

As if echoing our thoughts, Richard continued, "Margaret's chances aren't so hot, are they? But I'll get those organs for her—it'd be a pretty sorry thing if somebody who owns five TV stations couldn't orchestrate the necessary publicity. You know, sometimes in the middle of the night when I'm not too busy feeling sorry for Margaret, and her mother, and myself, I've spared a thought or two for the six people who won't get these organs Margaret needs, and I've felt pretty guilty that they'll die. But not guilty enough to stop what I'm doing, or to let Margaret go so those other people can live." He bit his lip and began to dig industriously at a patch of lichen with his thumbnail. Overhead a gull cried in the sunshine, and the green waters lapped the shore.

We didn't know what to say to him.[5]

A Variety of Views

There is a relationship between what justice demands for the six people who will die and the loyalty Richard Barrie is expected to show his daughter; one way to look at it might be called the "master" view: justice is simply the "master value," and values of loyalty must simply give way before it when they collide. If this is the right way to think, Richard is entitled to no more for his daughter than anyone else gets, and he certainly isn't entitled to six organs. Another interesting approach is the "assimilationist" view: loyalty is absorbed right into impartial justice. The idea is that impartialism permits everybody to favor certain people in certain instances—say, within families—at least up to a certain point. If this is correct, then Richard might be permitted to spend all the money and exert all the influence at his disposal—stopping short of lying, cheating, or stealing—to save his daughter. The world as a whole is a better place when fathers are permitted to favor their daughters. And a third orientation— the "spheres of justice" view—sees impartialism and loyalty as independent. Both are the primary guides to moral behavior in certain more or less distinct spheres of our lives; when they come into conflict with one another, that conflict might be resolvable with the aid of certain rules of thumb, or by the exercise of sophisticated moral judgment. For example, Richard would be entitled to exert influence on his daughter's behalf because the rules for families are different from the rules for business, but he shouldn't use his own TV stations to generate the appeals for organs because doing this mixes the sphere of business with the sphere of the family in ways that can't be justified.

While all these accounts contain valuable insights, we think that none of them will altogether suffice, and that it is time to search for an approach that doesn't subordinate, exclude, or restrict the scope of special loyalties, but rather reconceptualizes the idea of justice to include it. Instead of showing that loyalty to a dying daughter is locked in a losing battle with justice, as a "master" theory would, or that it is simply a local instance of impartial justice in general, as an assimilationist account might, what we really need to do is rethink what justice means in light of the moral importance of our loves and loyalties. Coming up with such a notion of justice is a big job and we can't do it all here, but we can provide at least an outline and a basic rationale for an understanding of justice that takes loyalty seriously. We can work out its implications for the problems illustrated in this book. But we're a little ahead of ourselves. First we need to show why the "master," "assimilationist," and "spheres of justice" views won't work.

The Master View

Contemporary discussions of justice often start with John Rawls, arguably the most significant living theorist in this area. In an uncharacteristically ringing phrase, Rawls has written, "Justice is the first virtue of social institutions, as truth is of systems of thought."[6] Rawls means that, no matter how comfortable, secure, or affluent a state's laws have made it, no matter how high the literacy rate or how low the infant mortality statistics, if the laws are unjust, they must be altered or abolished. Like truth, justice is an uncompromising virtue.

Here is the "master" view in all its glory. When we apply it to the social institutions that are the concern of this book, however, we have to ask the question, "Is justice really the 'first virtue' of families and medicine?" It's hard to see how the answer can be yes, particularly if we accept (as Rawls, for example, certainly does) that justice is a rigorously impartial idea. We might think that the first virtue of medicine is healing the ill, or comforting the suffering, and that the first virtue of families is forming and sustaining the particular selves inside them. If these social institutions perform their functions well, and if doing so means that they have to make small departures from what justice (impartially understood) would mandate, then perhaps that's a price worth paying. After all, healing, comforting, and sustaining selves are very significant moral goals in their own right.

The Assimilationist View

Perhaps the mistake is to see the virtue of justice and the virtue of favoritism as cut from different bolts of cloth, as potential competitors. Rather than place the values of family life and medicine in *competition* with the notion of justice, perhaps we can *assimilate* those values into it. After all, justice and favoritism are both social virtues—both necessary for communal living. And if the point of living in community with others is to satisfy as many people's interests as possible, then, as the philosopher James Rachels argues, the favoritism the parent shows his children and the physician shows her patients can be justified to the extent to which it provides what we all might impartially regard as a social benefit worth having: the satisfaction of significant human interests.[7]

Yet we've already seen something of the problem with this solution: if I love my children or serve my patients only to the extent that the general good demands, I am not truly loyal to them—when push comes to shove, and the greater good is not served by my favoring these people, I will abandon them and serve that greater good. Mrs. Jellyby, in Dickens's *Bleak House*, is a fine example of the triumph of impartiality; full of concern for the remote poor, she can see nothing nearer than Africa—including the needs of her own family. Despite its efforts to accommodate our intuitions about intimacy, the assimilationist view really makes Mrs. Jellybys of us all.

Perhaps this is less problematic for the doctor-patient relationship than it is for families: medicine's benefits, intimate though they are, might be conveyed even if a patient realizes that her interests do not weigh harder with the doctor than the interests of society as a whole.[8] The fact that Dr. Schliermacher is legally and morally allowed to reveal confidential information about Tom's father to the insurance company, for example, doesn't seem to have deterred Tom's father from going to the doctor. When all is said and done, Tom's father isn't looking primarily for loyalty and love from Dr. Schliermacher—he's looking for treatment for his heart disease. Still, even though the relationship is fundamentally instrumental, trust and loyalty are important to it because of the high premium we place on life and health and because the doctor has so much power. In families, on the other hand, the relationship is not finally instrumental: love and loyalty seem to be the major point. For that reason, the interests of family members have to count for more than society's interests to at least a marginal degree, or we can't say that love and loyalty are really present at all.

The Spheres of Justice View

Jamie and Dr. Schliermacher are both rightly reluctant to scuttle their loyalty to Tom's father altogether (on the Rawlsian grounds that to do so would not be impartial) or to favor him only up to the point that impartial justice allows (Rachels's argument). But the reasons for their reluctance are probably different, since familial relationships are different from medical ones. It is hard to come up with a unified account of moral favoritism that is equally illuminating for both, and accordingly the third option, dividing society up into different spheres operating on different principles, starts to look pretty attractive.

The political theorist Michael Walzer, who invented this view, thinks that structuring just institutions involves two large tasks. One is to work out what principles of distribution ought to govern the different spheres of life: business, politics, education, and so forth. This is accomplished by attending to the "social meaning" of the various goods involved in those spheres.[9] The second task is to make sure that the power and influence that stem from success in a given sphere don't trespass into other spheres: success in the sphere of money and commodities, for example, ought not to transfer directly into success in the realm of political power; being rich shouldn't guarantee being politically influential. Justice demands "nondominance": no sphere may lord it over any other.

Appealing as all this is, Walzer's version of justice has its own problems. The first is to figure out how the many spheres, with their different and autonomous conceptions of justice, can be coordinated to constitute a tolerably just social whole.[10] To do this, we might draw on the social meanings that characterize different spheres; perhaps there are ways in which, say, love and impartiality can influence each other without one dominating the other. For example, we might conclude that Richard Barrie is acting just exactly as a loving father ought, and that it's up to the transplant team or the United Network for Organ Sharing to set rules that would keep Margaret from getting more than her fair share of organs. But this brings us to the second problem, which is that contemporary Americans don't in fact agree about the social meanings that characterize the various spheres of our lives. Do we have a common understanding of the social meaning of organ sharing, for example? The dispute over organ sales suggests that we're not altogether clear about whether they ought to be assigned to the sphere of business.[11] And the deeper problem is, of course, that even when we do agree, we might be wrong. The social meanings we assign in different spheres can themselves be quite unjust.

Injustice in the Familial Sphere

This problem of social meaning is clearly illustrated in families, where there is an endemic form of injustice: that of gender. In U.S. families headed by a woman and a man who are married to each other, men do more paid labor and less domestic unpaid labor than women. But the air of equity that may seem to hover about this division is specious. For one thing, men do far less of the domestic unpaid labor than women even when the women are also working at paying jobs.[12] Furthermore, because of their greater access to paid labor, men earn more money, are paid at higher rates, and are in a better position to put together a collection of skills, experiences, and relationships that will allow them to continue to earn more than women. Beyond this, men are considerably freer both to contribute to the larger society (through artistic creation, scientific research, political leadership and the like) and to enjoy the satisfactions, excitements, prestige, and rewards that are on offer in that wider world.

These differences in earning capacity and range of opportunity are particularly significant in light of the fragility of modern marriage. Divorce is extremely common, as are its depressing consequences—men with reduced child care responsibilities enjoy sharply rising income, women with physical custody of children suffer from plummeting incomes. The pattern of "broken" homes merely recapitulates in more extreme form the patterns of "intact" families: husbands on average contributing fewer hours of paid and unpaid labor combined than do their wives; wives wielding less economic power, despite working longer hours.[13]

In the harsh light cast by these facts, the flaws in the traditional view—that families occupy their own sphere, separate from public life and falling under the sway of natural affections rather than the principles of justice—are glaringly obvious. Jamie is not merely tired and disgruntled at the end of an especially hard day—she is a victim of injustice, unfairly exploited because of her gender. It's not only that women have a harder time participating in the extrafamilial spheres—that it's more difficult for them to become captains of industry or orchestra conductors—it's also that within family life itself, as daughters, wives, and mothers, they are exploited by their husbands, sons, and fathers, and by their own mothers and daughters, too. The fact that Jamie loves and is loved by her family, and that we associate certain kinds of sacrificial meanings with the idea of motherhood, does not negate this conclusion. Such facts do, however, make it very difficult to figure out how to reform the situation.

Reform is further complicated by the smaller injustices that also bedevil families. For instance, Tom's father is grappling with the fact that the energy he once devoted to the projects that made his life meaningful is now waning. Having retired from the paying jobs that contributed to his sense of worth and importance, he feels—with some justification—that he is not as central to the family's enterprises as the younger generations are. Yet Jamie and Tom had no compunctions about expecting him to help rear the children, and there is a sort of implicit expectation that he'll help out with the kids' college tuition. After all, if Grandpa's no longer socially productive, he might as well make himself useful to the family.

Gender complicates all this; old women may be used to laboring within the home and so feel less dislocated than Tom's father, but both sexes are likely to resent it that within the family someone younger is calling the shots, and that they have been displaced from whatever positions of prestige and honor they once enjoyed. Even so, Tom's father loves his family and they love and are good to him; what would he gain if he insisted on his rightful share of familial power?

Injustice in the Medical Sphere

Medicine, too, has been considered a social sphere in which it's inappropriate to insist on justice. Yet physicians like those on Margaret Barrie's organ transplant team are custodians of immensely expensive resources, gatekeepers who not only control our access to these goods but control and create our desires for them. Ordinarily, being punctured, probed, irradiated, or sliced open are not high on the list of anybody's pleasures, but upon a physician's recommendation, we're willing to pay large sums for these privileges. Or, rather, we're willing to have large sums *paid* for the privileges: until recently, at least for middle- and upper-income people, insurance paid for virtually everything that the physician recommended. Out of the combination of a massively expensive, powerfully entrancing technology, a fee-for-service system, care provided almost free at the point of delivery, litigation pressures, the monopolistic character of the guild of physicians, and an aging population, has come a justice problem of the first magnitude: how do we keep medical costs, now amounting to a trillion dollars a year, from gobbling up all our resources when we also have other vitally important social needs?[14] We need to provide good schooling for our children, a vigorous industrial base, decent social services for the poor, a reasonable amount of aid to the arts, humanities, and sciences, environmental clean-up, repairs to the infrastructure, foreign aid. And at the same time, we need as a matter of justice to incorporate into the health system the nearly forty million Americans who at present have no reliable access to it. No cheap task, that.

Because doctors know what treatments are likely to benefit what patients, and this knowledge is the basis for the recommendations that generate the costs within the system, it seems they should be involved in deciding what's too expensive, so that money can be diverted elsewhere when fairness demands it. But asking doctors to keep an eye on social justice as they prescribe for their patients runs against the ancient moral tradition in medicine that the patient's interests come first. This is medicine's version of the struggle between the perspective of justice and the perspective of loyalty.

Medicine has another justice struggle as well. Although the number of women entering medical school is now for the first time roughly equal to the number of men, the profession is still rather inhospitable to women.

They are not promoted within hospital hierarchies as quickly or as often as men, they are not mentored as well, they are excluded from peer networks, and they are sexually harrassed by their male colleagues to a depressing extent.[15] Women physicians enjoy greater prestige and power than many of their less well placed sisters, but they practice their profession in a world arranged by men for the convenience of men. Nor does medicine discriminate solely against its own; its sexism is impartially directed toward the women it treats as well as the women doing the treating. In June, 1990, the General Accounting Office reported that despite a 1986 federal policy to the contrary, researchers had continued to exclude women from biomedical research. Although, for example, coronary heart disease is the leading cause of death in women, the effect of aspirin and low cholesterol diets was studied in male populations almost exclusively. Studies for treating AIDS frequently omit women, even though women are the fastest growing infected population. The litany here is a long one, culminating in what has become a classic example of sexist research: a pilot project conducted in the late 1980s on the impact of obesity on breast and uterine cancer—which was conducted solely on men.[16] Steps have been taken at the National Institutes of Health to remedy the problem of exclusion, but it has not gone away. Finally, because health insurance is linked to employment, and because many more women than men work in part-time or low-paying jobs that do not offer insurance benefits, many more women than men are denied access to the health care system.

Both spheres, therefore, have been assigned meanings that are internally unjust: families have a serious problem with age and gender justice, medicine has trouble with gender justice, cost containment, and inclusion. So the "spheres of justice" approach turns out to be just as inadequate for our purposes as the "master" and "assimilationist" views.

Justice within Intimacy

If the general theorists of justice can't help us, how about the people who have tackled the question of justice within intimacy head on? When it comes to families, Susan Moller Okin's *Justice, Gender and the Family* is widely regarded as the most ambitious contribution. Let's use her approach to think about Jamie's situation. Why, given the fact that many families enjoy common interests, shared lives, and deep loves, should so much be made of their precise patterns of distribution of effort? Why suggest that women and men in intimate relationships are actually in conflict? Okin's answer is that the commonality and sharing undoubtedly occurring in many families is no antidote to sexism, and that the women in families realize this and don't like it. Studies cited by Okin show that it isn't lost on women that they do more hours of work than men, nor that both men and women think the work women do is less interesting. Further, women resent both the fact that men do so little domestic work and that they are economically dependent on men. As Okin has pointed out, the domestic division of labor is not a matter of women's free consent to these arrangements: rather, "the major reason that husbands and other heterosexual men living with wage-working women are not doing more housework is that *they do not want to, and are able, to a very large extent, to enforce their wills.*"[17]

Apart from the wrong to women, this is a very serious distortion in one of the basic functions we have assigned to families: forming the moral character of the young. If **Virtues are learned at our mother's and father's knees,** how can families do a good job at teaching them when the labor and rewards of family life are so unfairly handed out on the lines of gender? How can families stand up against medicine's desire to use them to relieve some of its own problems in the just provision of benefits and burdens when its own distributions are so skewed from childhood on?

Okin has argued that ending sexism in the family requires "liberalizing" the family—which is to say, rearranging it according to a theory of justice based on consent and contract. She believes that moving toward justice in families will first require protecting those who are currently getting less than their fair share of the familial resources. For example, both partners to a marriage should have equal legal entitlement to all household earnings, and, if the marriage should end in divorce, both postdivorce households should enjoy the same standard of living.[18] But ultimately, when justice is fully realized, gender will not have any social significance. Okin calls for a society in which women and men share equally in the paid and unpaid work of society.

Okin is influenced by her creative appropriation of Rawls's work, and for that reason represents a kind of "master" approach. While her conclusions all seem, at first glance, extremely reasonable, her liberalization of the family is premised on a distorted view of the people inside it. A "liberalized" family is a family which is primarily contractual in character. To make the family more just, Okin believes, we will have "to destroy the mythical notion of it as a realm to which contractual thinking is inappropriate" and to push instead for contracts that distribute the family's burdens and benefits more fairly.[19] But as we've already argued, the contract model doesn't work very well for families, because it sees all the contracting parties as equally powerful, adult, rational, free agents, who can come and go independently and are answerable to nobody but their own consciences. This description doesn't even fit a man and a woman who are about to be married (and emotionally in thrall to one another), let alone a baby, a person suffering from senile dementia, or a teenager. Not only does the model fail to account for our responsibilities to *Family members,* who *are stuck with each other* (particularly children and parents), as we explained in Chapters Five and Six, it's also that it fails to notice that a family's characteristic functions *aren't replaceable by similarly (or better) qualified people*—another notion we've been at some pains earlier on in this book to explain. So it looks as if families are either going to be preliberal and unjust, or they will be just, but not really families any longer. Is there another alternative?

Moral Favoritism

We think so. Taking our cue from Iris Marion Young, among others, we see interpersonal relationships, rather than contractual distribution, as the appropriate subject of justice.[20] If you begin by taking account of the differences among members of the family—their different histories, degree of dependence on others, ability to contribute to the common welfare, level of education and understanding, special vulnerability and need—you might reply to Okin that in an unjust family, it isn't so much that individuals aren't (but should be) in equal bargaining positions as that certain people within the familial relationship have not been given their due importance. Because they are inside a system of intimacy, each person can be asked to contribute to the good of all according to his or her skills and capabilities, and each can expect to receive from the others what he or she requires to flourish. The problem for families is not to insist that each member go even-steven with every other from the same position of strength so much as to be vigilant that everyone is creatively included in the richness of family life—or at least that any distance or disaffection is the outcome of people's own free actions, rather than being forced upon them by virtue of their gender or age, their sexual orientation or their marital status.

The allocation of caring responsibilities in families should be seen as a question of equity, and the propensity to shovel inequitable amounts of caring labor on women should be explicitly faced (as should the needs of other family members for appropriate attention). But this can be done without assuming that all human relationships bear a fundamentally contractual character. Rather that endorse a principle of "equal split" of responsibilities between adults, for example, a more flexible kind of equity ought to be seen as the goal. Nobody should be stuck with more of the household drudgery than anyone else, but if one person's talents and tastes incline him to prefer auto maintenance to ironing, the drudgery might be divided along the lines that people find least onerous. As the philosopher Richard Aronson has pointed out, rigid adherence to an "equal split" rule may end up making everybody worse off.[21]

However, families need to realize that the assignment of labor between men and women, and of authority between old and young, is now far from equitable overall, that we all have a tendency to think that we are exceptions to these trends, and that our own patterns need to be subject to critical scrutiny. The adults and children in the family should explicitly realize and discuss the fact that everyone has inherited images of domestic life that act to exploit and exclude women, and that undermine the full and proper standing owed to the elderly and other family members. They need to recognize, address, and defuse the power of these images in their own families. These discussions shouldn't be seen as "negotiations" among rational, self-interested agents, but as efforts to improve the character of their joint life together.

This understanding of justice is inclusionary: everybody gets to participate, everybody pitches in. It is an understanding that uses the group's loving relationships to advantage, rather than discounting them or playing them down. It isn't altogether unlike the understanding of justice expressed in Jane Austen's Mansfield Park, where there is "a consideration of times and seasons, a regulation of subject, a propriety, an attention towards every body. . . . Every body had their due importance; every body's feelings were consulted."[22] Reconfiguring families to reflect justice of this kind will not be easy. It will require a clear sense on the part of everyone that things, as Jamie understands full well, are not as they ought to be in families; it will further require an understanding that the individual preferences of individual women and men in individual families are not the only considerations relevant.

This approach may seem naïve, and worse, tantamount to a concession to entrenched patterns of familial injustice. Is it really likely that any of this is going to help Jamie be less tired, less disgruntled, and less exploited at the end of the day? It is true that a great deal is left here to the good will of families, and in particular, to the willingness of women in families to stand up for themselves, of men to yield unfair privileges, and of everyone to cultivate a notion of respect for others that does not hinge on one's ability to generate a paycheck. But at some point, relying on good will and a sense of fairness is unavoidable if anything of familial privacy and intimacy is to be maintained. Short of government supervision, restructuring families to achieve justice must be a matter of relying on their members' common desire to do right by each other; this is as true of Rawls's approach (via Okin) as it is of ours. What we offer is a response to the theoretical claim that maintaining familial intimacy is incompatible with achieving familial justice. We've tried to show how in principle it's possible to achieve both; that is not to say that the achievement will be easy.

Jamie and her family have their work cut out for them, but at least there is a coherent goal for them to pursue. Before we turn to Dr. Schliermacher and his problem with justice, we need to consider one more point. Thus far, our discussion of caring labor within families has been focused on how it should be *distributed*. But familial justice also has to say something about how it may be *limited*. At what point may Jamie, or Libby and Deirdre, or anyoned else, for that matter, refuse to take on further tasks of care, even within their own family? How do we know when a family has reached its ethical "Plimsol line"—the point at which, no matter how you distribute the load, any additional weight will cause the whole ship to sink?

Obviously, the answer to this question will vary with the resources and situation of particular families, as we saw in the conflict Jeff faced between his promise to mother and the needs of his family in Chapter Five. The analysis there focused on the significance of "strong moral self-definition" for families; here, we presuppose that framework and try to extend it by an explicit consideration of justice issues.

TRANQUILIZERS IN THE SOUP

Gabe and Michael have often reflected that, while a three-generation, all-male household hardly lends itself to maximum domestic harmony, living with Michael's seventy-five-year-old dad, Joseph, has certainly added a rich tang to the family as a whole, and has brought an important extra dimension to the kids' lives in particular. Yet now that tang is turning decidedly sour: Joseph has grown increasingly nervous and increasingly—well, nasty. Gabe and Michael have seen this happen before, but last time the doctor prescribed tranquilizers that helped Joseph through the episode. This time he refuses to take them. "I don't trust doctors and I don't trust drugs," he maintains, "and besides, I don't want to walk around all the time feeling dull." But for Michael and Gabe and their three adopted children, his tantrums and complaints are sapping family life of much of its sweetness. Gabe is starting to think that things simply cannot go on this way, and Michael isn't far behind.

In retrospect, the tranquilizers seem magical to them. "Could we slip them in his soup, do you suppose?" Gabe asks his partner. "Otherwise, something's really going to have to give. You know, he needs help with a lot of things now, and it's just hell to try to do anything for him when he's being so godawful ornery all the time. Michael, we want him back."[23]

On the question of whether Jeff's mother ought to be placed in a nursing home, we stressed the significance of Jeff's decision as a contributor to the family's developing character; the promise he made his mother never to put her in a home was starting to exact a toll that he had not anticipated, and was being paid not by him alone, but by other members of the family. The family system itself was suffering. In the case of Michael's dad, the conflict hovers around the problem of deception, of not honoring the dignity of one family member, in order to secure a tolerable measure of tranquility for the whole. As in Jeff's case, Gabe and Michael might look to their past relationship with Joseph and the rest of the family, trying to discern morally relevant patterns they wish to endorse or to change. They might also look to the future, knowing that their decision in this case says something about who they take themselves and their family to be. But further help might still be welcome. To what extent does the way they *wish* to define themselves reflect how they *should* define themselves if justice is to be done?

A few distinctions might be of use. Some caring burdens within families are *mandatory*; that would seem to follow fairly directly from the idea of a group of people intimately concerned with and involved in each other's lives. Some burdens of care are *supererogatory*: they are praiseworthy, but a person is not open to censure for failing to assume them. That there is such a category would seem to stem from the idea that some part of your life belongs to you, even though your obligations to others are somewhat open-ended. And some caring demands may actually be *wrong* to undertake: those, for example, which seriously threaten a family's ability to engage in its other functions.

These distinctions, combined with the following rules of thumb, might be useful in helping family members to sort out the categories into which various caring demands fall. (For Gabe and Michael, one question to be answered before they resolve to put tranquilizers in the soup is whether the family has an obligation to care for Joseph in the way Joseph insists upon.) More generally, the rules include the following:

1. Familial caring burdens are just that—familial, not female.
2. Familial caring burdens are not altogether private—to some extent, they must be regarded as making a contribution to the social good, and hence, worthy of social support.

Rules One and Two attempt to situate caring burdens in a wider context. They point out some relevant implications of families' involvement in society: a warning that society's endemic sexism pervades families, and a reminder that society's interests are much affected, for good or ill, by what happens in families. The first rule has already been discussed; the second will become more significant in what follows. It should also be noted that these are expressly "balancing" rules, not "limit" rules. But they have "limit" implications. Sometimes, a family can't distribute its caring obligations equitably, perhaps because a chronically ill child thrives only with Mom's attention; no one else's will do. And society's estimation of its duties to contribute to such care are woeful. These "reality constraints" may push a family toward its own Plimsol line in practice, even if in principle there exists a better way of distributing burdens.

3. Familial caring burdens are only part of a whole range of needs families must serve, including supporting members' personal projects and tending the relationships among them. Families need to stay alert to the rest of the range.

4. Family caring burdens aren't all equally crucial—some are more significant than others, and individual family members may perceive their significance differently.

5. The meaning of particular acts of caring in particular family situations is variable. The people being cared for, as well as those caring, need to participate in the construction of that meaning. An appreciation of the general and specific goals of family life may be helpful in that construction.

Rules Three to Five suggest the need to situate a given burden of care within the particular context of particular families. They alert us to the importance of the fact that family members are always more than family members, and that the "extras" in a person's life aren't just whims but include projects of moral significance. They also emphasize that different kinds of caring have different kinds of significance: some things family members do for each other are perfectly well done by another qualified person; others are decidedly not. Some kinds of caring may be ambiguous in this respect, and discussion may be needed to determine where they fall. Different family members may, of course, have different ideas about what a given expression of care means. While some disagreements may be intractable, others might be resolvable, particularly if the members share a sense of what families in general are for, and what their family, in particular, is about. These questions of context are important, but they are not everything, which leads us to our next rule.

6. The age of the potential recipient of care may be taken into account only to the extent that it affects the length of time the burden of caring must be borne.

The point of rule Six is to give "everybody their due importance"; familial care that would be undertaken if Michael were the recipient may not be denied to Joseph merely because he's old and considered past it. It might be denied, however, if giving it seriously compromises the life-chances of another member of the family. Conversely, if Joseph were helpless and bedridden and wished to die at home, Michael and Gabe might well take his age into account and undertake this care on the grounds that it won't be for long, even though the same degree of care might justifiably be declined for a small child who is predicted to linger helplessly for many years. And this leads us to our injustice rule:

> 7. Burdens are unjust if:
>> (a) they importantly compromise the core functions of families;
>>> —or—
>> (b) they importantly compromise core projects of individuals; so long as
>> (c) good faith efforts to share, negotiate, and reduce burdens have been made.

This rule leaves a lot implicit, of course. It will be crucial to consider the relationship between the cost to the caregiver member in providing the care, and the cost to the sick member if the care is not provided. And once you have established that a burden of care is unjust, you may find that you must provide it anyway, because there is no one else to do it and *Family members are stuck with each other.* Suppose no nursing home is available or none can be paid for. Suppose the school district simply doesn't provide suitable alternative schooling for Johnny. Suppose the only options open to a paranoid schizophrenic teenager are living at home or living on the streets. In these cases, even though the burden is unjust, it would often be wrong to refuse it.

In general, all that can be said is that the degree to which the caregiver's other plans and projects may be compromised depends upon how dire the consequences of withholding care will be to the person in need, other things being equal. But let's suppose that the situation in Gabe and Michael's family is bad enough to compromise its viability. Joseph's refusal to take his tranquilizers has thrown the family's capacity for caring labor out of balance, producing an unjust distribution of familial resources. According to the rules, it's time for some good faith efforts here—but does putting tranquilizers in the soup unbeknownst to Joseph count as good faith?

One can imagine a couple of alternative strategies. One is simply to confront Joseph with the family's understanding of the limits of its ability to care, let him know that the limit is being pushed hard by his stubbornness in the matter of his drugs, and enlist his aid in seeking a solution that everyone can live with. This might be possible if Joseph were not irrational as well as irascible; if the strategy backfires, it could eventuate in a sharp break between him and the others. But even in the best of circumstances, it's risky; while limits are something we can all countenance abstractly, it's quite another thing when they threaten us concretely.

Another strategy is to spike the soup and then discuss with Joseph what was done and why. However, this attempt at "ex post facto" consent comes down, at best, to a matter of "moral luck": if Joseph is grateful and approving, the ploy with the soup was justifiable; if not, it was wrong.

But Joseph's consent is not the only moral matter at issue here. Michael and Gabe must also, in justice, consider the welfare of the rest of their three-generation household. As they go through the process of moral self-definition we described earlier, they'll need to get clear about whether they regard the sacrifices they've made as supererogatory, or whether it's more accurate to say that they had no choice but to do what they did. If their part in the moral story of their family has been to respond as they must rather than as they choose, they have a nonarbitrary reason for supposing that Joseph too has certain duties to the family: on this construal, Joseph's decision about the medication is not wholly his own. Involving him in a discussion of the issue after the soup has been spiked and he's a little more reasonable may be justifiable in this light.

We've presented a general way of understanding how justice should operate in families. We've also offered some rules of thumb to help Jamie and Tom and Michael and Gabe think about their families and their positions within them as they try to figure out the character and limits of their obligations and prerogatives. But what about the character of *medicine's* obligations and prerogatives? To look at this we need to turn back to Dr. Schliermacher.

Doctors, Patients, and Justice

The big justice question in health care is how to adjust the relationship between medicine and other parts of social life so that medicine can fairly provide its benefits to people without stinting education, environmental reform, and our other essential needs. Finally and fundamentally, it's a matter of reforming the structure of the health care institution as such. Would justice best be served by a Canadian-style, "single payer" system? Would a nationwide system of HMOs, engaged in "managed competition" with each other, be roughly as efficient, as inclusive, and more in keeping with our individualistic national culture? Or would some other kind of health care framework be better? These systemic questions are important, yet the system as a whole is not the only arena where change will have to occur. Much of the drama of achieving justice in medicine will go on within the smaller compass of the doctor-patient relationship.

Unlike familial relationships, doctor-patient relationships are at least quasi-contractual, and one of the most common laments about contemporary health care is that they are becoming less "quasi" and more "contractual" as the years go on. Roles and obligations, due in part to litigation pressures and in part to the new understanding of patient autonomy, are at least somewhat more explicit and more particularly focused than they used to be. But in the midst of what starts as an instrumental, economic, contractual relationship between strangers, a certain kind of intimacy must exist, and a certain form of trust must also flourish. The potential significance of what physicians and other health care providers may do for us, the physical and psychological openness that often must take place if we're to reap these benefits, require this intimacy and trust, and doctors have gone to elaborate lengths throughout the course of their profession's existence to secure them.

Their primary instrument for this job has been a moral undertaking: physicians since Hippocrates have pledged to focus on the good of their patients in a well-nigh exclusive fashion. This is clearly what drives Dr. Schliermacher. But ought it to? As Howard Brody notes, physicians have the power to "break the bank" in their efforts to do the best they can for their patients.[24] There is a litany here that bears repeating: as we hit the trillion-dollar level of annual health care spending in the U.S., we find ourselves spending at a rate that threatens other extremely significant social functions, leaves tens of millions of people outside the health care system, and, as a crowning irony, doesn't even seem to buy us care that is any better than that of many other, more frugal countries. The fact that the majority of spending decisions occurs at the hands of physicians therefore becomes inescapably important.

This argues strongly that physicians must take thought for more than patient welfare in making treatment decisions. The social welfare is too dependent on—or, to put it plainly, too threatened by—what physicians do, for physicians simply to "bracket" the wider impact of their decisions. But if physicians pay attention to the social cost of what they do, they are no longer putting the patient first.

As in families, so in medicine: both institutions are charged with the task of becoming more just, but doing it in ways that won't displace or even much disturb the particular forms of loyalty and attention that are key to their work. But the differences between the institutions can't be forgotten either: while Gabe, Michael, and Joseph have to work things out directly with each other, Dr. Schliermacher has the advantage of being able to rely on others to do the dirty work of saying no to patients. This possible compromise view is nicely expressed by the following argument, formulated (and criticized) by Brody:

> The physician is morally obligated to serve the patient first and foremost, not the interests of society or a health-care institution.
>
> When the physician is paid to deny services to patients to save the society or health care institution money, a conflict of interest is set up that constitutes unethical medical practice.
>
> It is undeniable, however, that the costs of medical care must somehow be constrained.
>
> Therefore, somebody other than the physician must act so as to deny certain categories of costly care to certain categories of patients.[25]

What this argument does, in effect, is to maintain boundaries between two "spheres of justice": the sphere of medical care needs to be kept distinct from the sphere of social accountancy. But there are costs to this way of doing business. Probably the largest cost is that a patient's access to medical services will be determined by individuals who aren't closely acquainted with the intricacies of her particular situation: decisions will be made on the basis of whether a patient falls into certain categories—categories that will surely be too broad to capture subtle but medically relevant differences among patients.

The implications are ironic: in an effort to protect the doctor-patient relationship as a means of assuring high-quality care, quality is actually threatened. Accordingly, the physician as patient advocate must respond to the decline in quality of care by using whatever channels of review and appeal there may be. It isn't hard to imagine that continual appeals of this kind will clog the channels, lead to lower quality of care, and frustrate legions of clinicians and administrators. But even if this grim scenario is avoided, there's reason to be disturbed. Justice's demands that costs be contained and access opened probably will require some loss of quality for some patients. We ought to be very careful, therefore, about building into the system anything that further threatens to erode quality.

What Brody proposes (and we concur) is that notions associated with intimacy, loyalty, advocacy, and so forth be extended into the realm of impartial justice: physicians—and perhaps nurse-practitioners—ought to have a role in determining what counts as "costworthy" care. Their traditional commitment to patient advocacy ought to influence the treatment recommendations they make for justice's sake. The upshot would be a system which neither indiscriminately offers every possible advantage to every patient no matter how marginal and expensive, nor withholds every debatable advantage from every patient, no matter how much a particular individual might benefit from it.

Brody has argued powerfully that the sense of inescapable conflict here is more apparent than real, that physicians have always had to make tradeoffs between what is best for one patient and other concerns (such as other patients, their own lives), and that the economic structure in which the majority of American physicians have practiced until now—the "fee-for-service" system—contains its own pressures, which are quite capable of distorting the physician's allegiance to the good of her patient.

This last point highlights a particularly fascinating part of Brody's thinking. Himself a family practitioner, he believes that much of our concern about patient interests being underserved in systems that pay attention to cost comes from adopting the perspective of the subspecialist, who tends to believe that more is better, where "more" is typically high-tech, high-cost intervention. If, on the other hand, we adopt the perspective of the primary-care health provider, with her stress on "high-touch" over "high-tech" care, her interest in discussion, education, negotiation, and very importantly, her concern to avert the damage to the patient that may ensue from the very treatment itself, it becomes clear that more is not always better.

Of course, sometimes it *is* better—decidedly so. But the position doesn't rest simply on a "less is more" philosophy. Using Brody's approach, any denial of access to test or treatment would proceed from a careful analysis of the particular patient's position and occur within an open discussion. The net result might not only be the kind of fiscal responsibility justice demands, but could also keep the patient from unneeded interventions—a very distinct individual benefit, and one that could enhance, not diminish, overall health.

It's important to note that Brody is talking about using health providers as "gatekeepers" or "case managers" within a system whose foundation is a general concern for justice. Patients and the public generally would understand that physicians were taking a role in helping to determine what counts as costworthy care; physicians would be reimbursed in ways that undercut neither their ability to perform justly in that role nor their commitment to patient interest.

This is a powerful picture. However, Dr. Schliermacher, not yet converted from the traditional Hippocratic faith, still has an arrow or two left in his quiver. It is all very well, he might say, to point out that doctors have always had conflicts of interests to deal with, but some of those simply can't be eliminated: we could scarcely have a system of celibate, single-purpose physicians, each of whom serve only one patient. Nor could we expect them to work for free. Any system for paying physicians will contain some incentive to over- or undertreat. But why add concern for social justice to the already existing conflicts of interest? If you stop to think about it, many doctors haven't handled even the old conflicts so terribly well. Why are we confident they will do better with the new? And finally, wouldn't Brody's gatekeeping require a radical reconfiguration of society? As things now stand, we have no idea what would happen to the money a socially conscientious physician might save by not prescribing "uncostworthy" care. It could just as easily end up being spent on potato chips as on education for inner-city kids.

We think Dr. Brody has the better of the argument with Dr. Schliermacher. The stakes are so high that doctors simply must start taking the economic consequences of their decisions into account. It would certainly be preferable if this could be done in a "closed system," where every dollar saved on marginally beneficial health care went to buy something substantially beneficial, like better prenatal care for poor women. But it isn't clear that this is an absolute moral requirement. We set a limit on what we're willing to spend on the safety of cars and high rise buildings, after all, without insisting that the money we save be spent on making other cars or other buildings safer than they otherwise would be. What is clear is that when a part of the system goes fiscally out of control, it's irresponsible to ignore the problem. Neither physicians nor patients cease to be citizens when they assume roles in the medical system: what significantly threatens all of us is a responsibility for each of us.

The fundamental point here is that all advocacy is advocacy within limits: while a nurse may try her utmost to convince the other members of the health care team that a particular patient needs better pain control, she can't just steal morphine and administer it herself; while Richard Barrie can buy medical care for his dying daughter, he arguably shouldn't be using his own television stations to elicit six organs for an operation that's almost certainly not going to succeed. What's needed here is a vision of justice that can provide guidance to both physicians and patients, a kind of guidance that will set mutually comfortable limits on advocacy, that will eventually make giving patients streptokinase or even aspirin rather than t-PA as much a matter of course as not stealing morphine for nonprescription use.

In our discussion of justice within families, we stressed the importance of overcoming the marginalization of women and other family members, of bringing them fully into the intimate association. If this is the spirit in which we approach the internal reform of families, then they can become just (juster, at any rate) without turning into an adversarial cluster of rights-seekers. If we want something similar to happen in medicine, we need the same kind of elements we identified earlier: a clear sense of what justice in "bedside rationing" would look like, and a clear sense of the spirit in which it should be undertaken.

This leads us to underscore a point implicit in the story of Richard and Margaret Barrie: it isn't physicians alone, but rather physicians, patients, and their intimates—typically, their families—who must come to practice responsible medicine. Thus, opening up medicine to the full significance of the importance of justice is not unlike the bioethical revolution that began a quarter of a century ago, when serious attention began to be paid to respect for patient autonomy. Patients and their intimates need to know that considerations other than their own best chances for marginal benefits are relevant to choice of care, and they need to lend their own authority to the process of denying themselves such care.

If patients and families don't participate in the project of making the health care system more just, they are likely to be marginalized by the policymakers. They need to remain ends in themselves if they are to avoid becoming simply means to the ends of society. If they take care to include themselves in the decisions that will produce a more just system, then any bedside rationing that goes on in effect occurs in public, within the context of a shared understanding of what the stakes are, with opportunity for discussion, negotiation, and compromise. In this way, the moral nature of the physician-patient relationship is preserved. All those involved in the healing relationship will understand it as a relationship of special loyalty and trust, but will also see that this loyalty has its limits, as all loyalty does. The broad outline of those limits will have gained public acceptance, so when treatment is limited, this won't be felt as "outsiders telling doctors what to do," but a natural part of the doctor-patient relationship.

Is it realistic to hope that patients, their families, and doctors will ever come to share this rosy vision? In particular, will members of our community who have been socially marginalized—African Americans, Native Americans, people living in poverty—accept that they have enough stake in the well-being of the community as a whole to regard even minimal sacrifices for its welfare as in their interests? And even if they or other community members could bring themselves to accept the need for medical spending limits in theory, would they be able to stick to it if their own interests are involved? Would Richard be willing to do only all he ought, rather than all he can, to care for his daughter?

What needs to be done to get families and individual patients to answer "yes" to questions of this sort is to engage them not simply in the process of bedside rationing, but in the process of rationing generally, at a systemic level. Insofar as people participate in the debate about this issue in the growing "health decisions" movement and in other such arenas, they will come to see more clearly just how our communal life is threatened by the continuation of a medical system that doesn't count costs and excludes fifteen percent of the population. They will come to see that their own access to good care requires priority setting at all levels. While it's unrealistic to suggest that citizens at the grassroots level should have responsibility or even substantial input into fine-grained medical policy decisions, the broad outlines of the medical system and its place with respect to other social goods should be decided by everyone through participation in a democratic process.

Such participation at the most general level will help people understand the advantages of rationing at the bedside level, and will allow them to commit themselves to it in a cool and reflective moment. Tom's father will experience moral dissonance if he believes in theory that solid, no-frills health care for everyone is better than luxury care for some and no care at all for others, but then demands t-PA for himself after his next heart attack. But grassroots participation might also empower Gabe and Michael to resist illegitimate encroachments on their family by a health care system eager to shift its burdens and costs somewhere else in the economy. It is to both of these matters—expecting families to bear too much and too little of the burden—that we now turn.

DON'T TELL SIS

Carlos is a twenty-one-year-old Hispanic man who had suffered gunshot wounds in his stomach in gang violence. He was uninsured, and his stay in the hospital was somewhat shorter than might have been expected, but otherwise unremarkable. It was felt that he could safely complete his recovery at home. Before leaving the hospital, Carlos told his physician that he was infected with HIV. Tests confirmed his report.

Carlos's attending physician recommended a daily home nursing visit for wound care, but Medicaid refused to fund nursing visits because there was someone at home who could provide this service—Carlos's twenty-two-year-old sister, Consuela.

Consuela was willing to do the wound care if someone would show her how. Since their mother's death when she was twelve, Consuela had tried to be mother to her brother and their younger sister. Carlos had no objection to Consuela's caring for him, but he insisted absolutely that she was not to know that he was HIV positive: despite their closeness, he had never told her that he was actively gay. It wasn't so much that he feared her knowing, although that would have been bad enough. What he feared even more was that his father would find out. The father, like many men of his culture and class, was intensely homophobic.[26]

This case is often used to focus discussion on the scope of a patient's right to medical confidentiality. But a subtheme running powerfully through it is the exploitation of women's labor in the family to supplement the health care system. As Marcia Angell, executive editor of the *New England Journal of Medicine,* put it in her commentary when this case first appeared in the *Hastings Center Report:*

> I can't help feeling that this young woman has already been exploited by her family and that the health care system should not collude in doing so again. We are told that since she was twelve, she has acted as "mother" to a brother only one year younger, presumably simply because she is female, since she is no more a mother that he is. Now she is being asked to be a nurse, as well as a mother, again presumably because she is female.[27]

This is not to allege that physicians or hospital administrators are holding guns to women's heads. But it does suggest that the tradition that justice isn't applicable in families is far from dead. In fact, the tradition isn't even fatally ill; medical reforms themselves seem to be pumping new life into it.

Let's suppose that Carlos was not HIV-positive, and that his sister was simply being asked to participate in his wound care in a situation that presented her with virtually no physical risk. Is Angell's point about the demands on her wedded to Carlos's serostatus? Is she exploited only if information is kept from her that might affect her decision to provide the care? Or would Angell's point still hold if Carlos were free of any infectious disease, and the only question were whether it was proper to withhold Medicaid funding for a nurse if there was someone in the home capable of providing the care? And if such care is exploitative, should medicine conclude that it's okay to go along with Medicaid unless the family is *particularly* exploitative? Or are all families so exploitative of women that no such shifting of further care to their shoulders is warranted?

In our opinion, even if Carlos weren't HIV-positive, Angell would still have a point. Shifting heavy-duty patient care onto families makes it harder for them to redistribute their own burdens and benefits in a way that no longer marginalizes the women who live inside them.

Still, one of the great sources of hope for restructuring medicine is to "despecialize" it: high-priced subspecialists should not do what family practice docs can do; family practice docs should not do what nurse practitioners can do; and (by parity of argument) professionals should not do what family members—the real primary health care providers—can do. If "despecialization" of this sort makes the health care system more just because it curbs overpricing, it might be sensible to ask whether care can be shifted from hospitals to homes in ways that do no (or only very little) harm to patients, and that do no (or only very little) harm to families.

Cost is not the only injustice in the health care system that shifts problems from hospitals to homes. Consider organ donation again. Because the system of organ retrieval in the United States is somewhat hit-or-miss, perpetuating a chronic shortage, and because the system of organ distribution is subject to unfair pressures (as when the media publicize Margaret Barrie's or some other "poster child's" need for an organ, or an experimental protocol allows a patient to jump the queue, or, perhaps, when an organ goes to the sickest person instead of someone who might benefit more greatly from it), many people die before a suitable organ becomes available. This means that when a family member needs a live organ that can be obtained by live donation, there may be considerable intrafamilial pressure to donate—pressure Richard Barrie certainly felt. The biological relationship among family members can sometimes produce a better match between donor and recipient, and that is an additional reason why family members make good donors. But if the pool of available organs were larger, a match could more easily be obtained without having to resort to live donation, which demands a far greater sacrifice on the part of the donor than cadaver donation does. In effect, the family is forced to make up for the shortcomings of the organ allocation system.

Part of what's needed here is for families to be able to challenge these demands, to have the right of appeal when extraordinary sacrifices would threaten their ability to meet other goals. As one of these goals is justice, a reasonable ground of appeal should be that the burdens cannot be equitably divided, and would fall on one person in such a way that her basic projects were severely compromised. But it would be better, of course, if the forces that cause such unjust concentration of burdens were addressed.

If society regards it as appropriate that more medical care go on inside homes, then other spheres of society must be willing to make available the resources to meet this burden. For example, places of business ought to allow greater flexibility in their employee's schedules to permit them to care for their sick. Corporations ought to do this on purely self-interested grounds: the point is to slow the growth of health care spending, which is making American goods less competitive in international markets. But it is also true that businesses depend upon the support provided by families in countless other ways. If they suffer costs or inconveniences in helping families to be better places, that can be regarded as a kind of tax in support of an infrastructure that is essential to business. Similarly, as organ transplantation has become a standard medical technique routinely offered by health care providers and routinely paid for by insurance companies, society needs to do a better job of making organs available so that the responsibility for supplying them doesn't fall so heavily on the patients' families.[28]

Finally, families should recognize their own stake in the decision to assume burdens. We don't mean to suggest that these are entirely a matter of decision, as we hope we've already made clear. Some burdens are simply a part of what it is to live in a family. But our analysis suggests that too many such burdens, unjustly distributed, threaten basic family functions of great moral significance. While it's hard (although not impossible) to see family members refusing each other essential help on this plea, the society in which families and health care institutions are nestled must begin to take more seriously the disasters that can ensue when a family's capacity to look after its own is drastically overloaded.

But the negotiations have to go both ways. We have discussed the moral commitment of physicians to their patients, commitments which place pressure on medicine's efforts to assume a just place within the overall distribution of resources. We have discussed the tendency of medicine to resolve its problems by reallocating caring burdens to the home, thus making its struggles with issues of gender and intergenerational justice even harder. Now it's time to discuss the family's tendency to demand more of medicine than it can justly give in the treatment of patients—the final link in a feedback loop that must be interrupted.

NEVER SAY NEVER

Jack Rosenbaum was twenty years out of medical school; he was hardly a *naïf*. Still, he never could face these situations without a sinking feeling in the pit of his stomach. Another shot-up kid caught at the edge of death by a too-successful EMT and a respirator, deep in a coma, never going to get any better. Another family who simply couldn't believe that such a thing could happen to their son, simply couldn't believe that all these high-priced docs and machines couldn't do something to give their boy back to them, simply couldn't believe that life could be so pointless.

He walked into the hospital's sun parlor, where the parents were waiting, and sat down with them. They were nice people—way out of their element, careworn, hardworking.

"Mr. Harris—Mrs. Harris. How are you?"

"Is Terry any better?"

"Well, that's what I wanted to talk to you about. I'm awfully sorry, but I think it's time we considered changing our goals for Terry's care. By now it's clear that the respirator isn't going to help him get any better. He's just going to hang on in a coma until he gets an infection we can't wipe out and he dies of that. What we're doing now isn't really worth anything to him."

There were several moments of silence while it started to sink in. Jack was braced for their response. Were they going to be resigned to the inevitable?

"Don't say that. It's keeping him alive. There's always some hope while he's alive."

"I really don't think so, Mrs. Harris. I hate to remember how many cases like Terry's I've been through. People who are as badly hurt as he is just can't get better. We don't have the ability to fix the damage to his brain."

"But you can't be sure, can you? Not absolutely sure that he won't wake up?"

Jack hesitated. "Not absolutely sure, no," he admitted. "But I am sure there's nothing more we can do to make it happen. It really would be a miracle, and if a miracle is going to happen, it'll happen whether we take him off the respirator or not."

"Then leave him on. It's not hurting Terry, is it?"

"No, but—"

"All right, then—aren't you really saying that his life isn't worth your time and effort? That it's too expensive to try to save his life? It's the only life he's got, Doctor. He needs that respirator."

What might help communication between doctor and family here? Increasingly, clinicians and theorists are saying that certain kinds of intervention are without any medical point, and that they are the proper professionals to identify such situations as "medically futile," as a matter of professional integrity. In this view, leaving a patient like Terry on a respirator indefinitely is not, properly speaking, an appropriate use of medicine, even though it's done with medical tools and skills. It's a little like someone coming to a doctor and requesting that a healthy leg be amputated because he finds it sexually satisfying. A surgeon might well know how to do this, but she is not practicing medicine if she does.

The problem with this analysis, however, is that the analogy doesn't hold. While amputating a healthy leg is indeed an idiosyncratic notion of what a proper medical goal should be, extending life is not. What the doctor in Terry's case is doing is only futile if the outcome—the continuation of Terry's life in a coma—is worthless. And this is a judgment that doctors have no special expertise to make. In this instance, the agreement between the provider and the recipient of care that forms the basis for authorizing any medical intervention—the agreement about what's worth doing—has evidently broken down.[29]

But if the *doctor* can't appeal to a notion like "medical futility" to excuse him unilaterally from any further duty to this patient, we can make *social* judgments that the benefits of health care are too low to justify their expense, since the money they absorb could be spent on benefits of greater value. To judge that a comatose life is without value is an absolute judgment, one that's sure to be controversial in a pluralistic society. But to judge that a comatose life is less worthy of support than a sentient life is a comparative judgment to which we all adhere—indeed, if someone were indifferent to the choice between a life in a coma and a life of ordinary activities and abilities, we would have a hard time understanding why she gets out of bed in the morning.

In situations of this sort, where the ability of family and physician to negotiate together has apparently broken down, the first response ought, of course, to be an attempt to restore effective communication. Perhaps the family is calling for continued treatment simply because it hasn't come to grips with the relevant facts. Perhaps its members no longer trust the professionals with whom they deal. Perhaps they have reasons of their own for thinking that their loved one has a better than average chance of improvement. And perhaps any and all of these reasons for resisting professional advice to shift treatment goals are open to change. But if family and physician are simply unable to negotiate a satisfactory resolution of their differences, then explicit professional guidelines on the provision of care, preferably ratified by some sort of public input, should be available which provide a morally defensible background for the withdrawal of life-sustaining care.

The real question for families is what they ought to be aiming at in situations of this sort. How should they balance the interests of their loved ones against the interests of others? For Terry's parents the issue is quite straightforward. The boy's chances of benefitting in any way that he or his parents would recognize as improvement—apart from simply staying biologically alive—are virtually nil. The Harrises are not committed to vitalism, the view that life of any kind at any price is always better than no life at all. They do seem committed to saying that even an infinitesimal chance of recovery is worth any amount of social resources. If their boy has even one chance in a million of recovery, they don't want to take the risk of losing that one chance.

But if they were to look to their own practices as a family, to the patterns of value they have lived by for years, they would see that they have never insisted that everything be done in order to *avoid* an infinitesimal chance of a very *bad* outcome. It makes no more sense to insist that everything be done in order to *court* an infinitesimal chance of a very *good* one. It's not likely, for instance, that the Harrises have ever invested all their life's savings on lottery tickets, on the off-chance that they might win. Do they honestly think it's all right to invest other people's money on an equally bad chance of winning a miracle for Terry?

Of course, Terry's mom and dad may not be in a position to be reflective and analytical about this choice: they are operating out of shock, out of a crushing sense of loss both of their child and of any idea that the world is a decent place, and perhaps out of guilt and shame. But as they work through these feelings, a place for them to go back to is their own

217

practice as a family, where high-stakes gambling was off limits, and self-ishness was considered a major weakness. If they can work their way back to this understanding of how their family at its best faces crises, they may be able to realize that in letting Terry go, they aren't failing him in any way. And if the Harrises can achieve this kind of moral clarity in their extreme situation, they can stand as a sort of model to other families, such as Margaret Barrie's, who feel the inclination to push not only medicine but the larger society to do "everything" for their loved ones.

Families, Medicine, and Society

We opened this chapter with the image of a commuter into New York City, who sees in her fifty-minute ride not only the immense beauty of the Hudson River but also the immense variety of the disorder and injustice that plague human societies. Both sights are commonplace and at the same time overwhelming; the Hudson's beauty continues despite what we do to it, and so do the city's injustices. But the injustices in families and in medicine, though deeply rooted and pervasive, occur in contexts where there is often also altruism, good will, caring. Here, at least, we ought not to feel overwhelmed. Here indeed we need to do better, not only because we should always try to do better, but because of the relative tractability of the problem. If the institution of medicine and the institution of the family are like two enormous glaciers whose rubbing together produces friction, then a strategy for getting them to fit together more comfortably is to reconfigure them. A careful application of justice, understood in all the senses we have explored, would go a long way toward that reconfiguration.

Coda

Medicine, Families, and Other Sources of Identity

FROM ITS LEGENDARY HIPPOCRATIC PAST TO ITS PROBLEMATIC "managed care" present, medicine has prided itself on the patient-centered character of its ethics. But patients, as we have been at some pains to point out, exhibit a very persistent tendency to come stuck to families of some sort or other. Medicine hasn't been able to escape dealing with these attached people. Family members are not patients, yet professional health care givers haven't been able to dismiss them altogether.

It would be somewhat surprising, then, if medicine's moral traditions were completely innocent of any acknowledgment of families. In this coda, we want to suggest that there is at least a hint that medicine's traditional moral self-understanding has included some grasp that families matter, and even (although this is less certain) of why they matter. What is interesting about this hint is that it may serve as a connection between medicine's past—a perpetually invoked source of its self-understanding—and medicine's future—a future in which morally important *cultural* differences among patients will become increasingly visible and will resist suppression.

219

Whether medicine has had some inkling of the significance of intimate connection or not, we will end this book by arguing that its encounter with a multicultural future can best be guided by the greater sophistication about families for which we've been calling. That is, families can serve as an avenue of approach to the issues of multicultural diversity that medicine, at least in the United States, has had to begin to take seriously.

Ancient medical moral codes haven't had a great deal to say about matters of familial intimacy, but a sensitivity about giving scandal—a social notion bound up with the ways we structure our intimate lives—seems to be a popular theme. For example, the "Five Don'ts" of Chinese medicine, formulated in the Ming Dynasty, advise the doctor not to see certain classes of female patients except in the presence of another person, and to reject even impure thoughts when attending "someone's mistress." Although these warnings may have more to do with preserving the doctor's status as a trustworthy and therefore employable professional than with any more high-minded concerns, it's also possible that they reflect an understanding of the importance of not upsetting the household by disturbing the relationships of intimacy inside it.

The cards are laid out a bit more plainly on the table in the Hippocratic tradition, which forbids engaging in sexual relationships with members of the patient's family. The Oath of Hippocrates commits the physician, in "whatever houses he may enter," to remain "free of all intentional injustice . . . in particular of sexual relations with both female and male persons, be they free or slaves." Now, "female and male persons" could, of course, refer solely to patients. And even if one took the phrase to refer to all inhabitants of the sick person's home, one could of course be cynical, and see in the prohibition only the fear that the physician would lose social and professional clout if he were found *in flagrante delicto* with one of the servants. But one could also see in the passage some acknowledgment of the way in which a violation of the familial order is felt by patients as a violation of the self, and therefore of patient trust. And here is where one can pick up the hint that medicine—particularly during that time in which it took its services into the patient's household—was importantly concerned with trying to spare that household from unnecessary disruption due to its encounter with a force both alien and, in its own way, intimate.

These days, house calls seem about as distant from us as the age of Hippocrates or the Ming Dynasty. Now, of course, medicine typically invites patients, and perforce their families, into its own houses. But the concern we have attributed—perhaps too generously—to ancient medicine about minimizing disruptions to the family is still in operation, even though the issues are really far more complex than a simple prohibition against having sex with a patient's intimates would indicate.

What's really at stake when the patient finds herself in the foreign world of contemporary medical care is the disruption of the flow of resources that families offer their own: the resources of care and the processes for maintaining the patient's sense of self. Forestalling this disruption will require not merely that health care professionals avoid easily definable activities such as sexual relations and impure thoughts where the patient's family is concerned, but an active, thoughtful, and rather iconoclastic shift in orientation. The task will be to set the traditional understanding that households are not to be disrupted any more than is necessary into a richer context—that of appropriately acknowledging the full particularity of patients—and to see that the kind of attention to families that we've called for are a large and essential part of this richer context.

Medicine deals in its day-to-day practice with people of all kinds—all races and ethnicities, genders and sexual orientations; different classes and age groups and different networks of kith and kin; varying degrees of illness, anxiety, and damage. But despite this great variety, there's a persistent temptation to see patients in the light of the leading model of moral agency that so permeates our culture—the image of the rational, calculating self-asserter, whose source of moral direction is nothing more than his own free choice, and whose important relationships are all chosen, quasi-contractual, and have nothing to do with his own fundamental identity.

So, inside every elderly and disabled woman of color suffering from cervical cancer, inside every six-year-old child grappling with her HIV infection, inside every Native American woman dying of breast cancer there is supposed to be a competent and self-interested, white, middle-class man of European origin, with a good grasp of medical realities and a firm handle on his own values, struggling to get out and negotiate appropriate treatment with his caregivers.[1] For that matter, this same competent and independent fellow lurks inside every white middle-class male patient as well. Treatment directives, durable powers of attorney for health care, and, when they fail, the directives of family members or friends (who know and love the patient intimately and are at the same time detached and disinterested) are the means currently in use to unearth this true self from its prison of infirm flesh. And when all these means are unavailable, or useless, we try to stare directly at that image of the rational self-asserter, and discern what it is that the generic reasonable person would find in his own best interest.

There are good reasons why this model has such a tremendous grip on our moral imaginations even in medicine, where that competent, self-possessed man inside such a variety of anxious and vulnerable bodies can be so hard to see. Isn't the job this man is doing of the utmost importance, helping families and caregivers to tailor treatment to what the patient really wants for herself or himself, independently of the irrelevant values of others? And what would we do without him, anyway? If we don't have an ideal of the reasonable patient as a touchstone by which to measure the actual patient's decisions, and still more, against which to assess the decisions of those who may serve as her proxies, how will we ever be able to discern the authoritative judgments, which we ought to respect, from the ill-made, "incompetent" ones, which we ought to challenge?

Through the course of this book, we have tried to dethrone this image of the self-possessed man, because he seems so distant from the way in which real people are so often enmeshed in webs of intimate connections, and because catering to him undermines the medical impulse to protect and strengthen those relationships of intimacy that contribute to a patient's well-being. The fact that we are situated as people so often tend to be, in a field of back-and-forth influence with others whose good is so caught up with ours, contributes to our identities and to our fundamental welfare. The myth of the ideal reasonable man is simple and powerful and has had very important benefits, but if medicine is to serve people better as we move into the next millennium, it has to wean itself from this one-dimensional picture of what humans are and wherein their good resides, just as patients must surrender an image of medicine that is too simple and too powerful.

When we come to grips with the character and value of familial intimacy in all its varieties we will have contributed to the job of getting a more accurate and at the same time still useful image of the patient with whom medicine works. But our relationships with our families aren't the only sources of moral complexity, nor the only ways in which our selves are shaped and supported. We construct our identities from our cultural heritage, our ethnicity, our class, our gender, our religious commitments, our generation, our sexuality, and the various particular abilities and vulnerabilities of our bodies. An ethics that tries to illuminate the relationship between medicine and the rest of society out of a growing awareness that the relationship is set in a multicultural, pluralistic world will need to think through all of these ways in which identities are shaped, and figure out how to do them appropriate honor.

A striking example of failure in this respect occurred recently in a Western hospital, where a Native American man was receiving treatment. Members of his community—family and friends—gathered in his room and conducted a ritual of healing, according to the traditions of the tribe. Unfortunately, hospital staff lacked the ability to see the ritual as allied therapy, or even as anything other than drunken and threatening behavior; they called hospital security and had the patient's family thrown out of the hospital.

How could this have been prevented? One possibility is some sort of ad hoc approach to cultural sensitivity, in which staff are alerted to specific kinds of behavior which are to be allowed for specific kinds of people: reasonable accommodations must be made for Native Americans to perform healing rituals, for people from southeast Asian backgrounds to have rice in their meals, and so forth. But a better approach would be more general, and flows naturally out of the sensibilities we have been encouraging here. Just as families serve as conduits to the individual patient's self and values, so they can serve as conduits in the other direction—as avenues to the patient's culture. Families stand as mediators between the whole range of cultural particularities that form a person and the expression of these particularities in that person's interaction with nurses, doctors, and other helpers.

In the exploration we've undertaken here of ways in which a more sensitive view of families can alter and improve medical practice, we have also been exploring how the particularities of people can make their presence felt more vividly within health care settings. One final story shows how these themes run together.

MRS. SHALEV AND HER DAUGHTER

Mrs. Shalev is now eighty-three years old. She was born in Poland and escaped to the United States in the earliest years of the Second World War. Mrs. Shalev adapted pretty quickly to Brooklyn, raised a family there, and developed a reputation as a quick-witted person who was meticulous about most things in her life, including her health and her medical care.

Two years ago, Mrs. Shalev suffered a serious stroke. Since then, she has spent a good deal of her time in hospitals and nursing homes, always carefully attended by her daughter, Becky Putnam, whose home Mrs. Shalev had shared for the five years just before her stroke.

Mrs. Shalev is now back in the hospital, with a long list of serious problems. Her physicians regard her situation as "short-term survivable, long-term terminal." But she still has periods of lucidity, and her daughter (and to a lesser extent, her son-in-law) is still deeply involved in her care.

In the opinion of the team treating Mrs. Shalev, her daughter may in fact be too deeply involved. Ms. Putnam is particularly concerned about the amount of pain medication that her mother is getting. Both Mrs. Shalev's kidneys and her liver are compromised, and Ms. Putnam believes that large doses of morphine or other powerful analgesics might cause further harm to those organs, thus hastening her mother's death. Further, the analgesics rob her mother of the little capacity for relationship that she has left—in particular, the ability to recognize her daughter's presence.

At the same time, Mrs. Shalev has developed a number of serious pressure sores from being bed-bound so long. Some of these are bad enough that bone tissue shows through. She needs regular changes of the dressings on these sores, and this is apparently quite an uncomfortable procedure. How uncomfortable, no one can really tell, but she certainly reacts negatively to them, moaning and trying to pull away.

The treatment team also feels that it's time to start rethinking the goals for Mrs. Shalev's care more generally. She is currently undergoing a number of invasive treatments, none of which have any real chance of making her any better; the best they can do is spin out her life just a little longer. Some of the physicians involved in her care have been heard to utter the word "futility," and the nurses in particular are very concerned that the aim of Mrs. Shalev's treatment be to keep her as pain free as possible so that she can end her life in dignity and comfort.

Ms. Putnam has a very different view of the matter. While she doesn't deny that her mother faces a grim outlook, she does believe that the growing consensus of the treatment team is inappropriate, to put it mildly. She insists that her mother continue to receive aggressive, life-sustaining treatment, and that the analgesics be minimal. During one care conference, she exclaimed, "Where we come from, we find it offensive that you insist on discussing withdrawal of life support—we have never even talked about these things among ourselves!"

This position is rapidly driving the treatment team crazy. The call goes out to the hospital's ethics committee in hopes that some strategy for changing Ms. Putnum's mind can be worked out. Failing that, perhaps there's a way of getting her out of the decisionmaking loop. As one nurse puts it, "While I respect the unique perspective of the family, there have to be limits. I feel as though I'm being forced to participate in the abuse of a vulnerable adult."[2]

In this case, we see a clash between the "reasonable, competent, self-interested man" whom the treatment team sees inside Mrs. Shalev, and the vision of the meticulous, *shtetl*-educated, Holocaust escapee, the wife of Abner, the mother of four daughters, who is preserved by Ms. Putnam. It seems unlikely that any reasonable, competent, self-interested person would want to undergo continual affronts to her dignity for the kind of life that medicine can offer Mrs. Shalev; it seems wildly implausible that any reasonable, competent, self-interested person would put up with considerable and quite unnecessary pain in order to lessen the chance of dying a little sooner than otherwise. If a family member insists on continued medical care and restricts pain control—particularly if, as in this case, there has been no discussion of the issue in explicit terms, no clear expression of preference and transfer of authority—there's something very wrong going on. There must be some kind of inability to let a loved one go, some kind of guilt mechanism working, perhaps some strange desire to punish Mother for dying or for some other imagined wrong.

But the daughter herself provides a window into the story that Mrs. Shalev has been living out, as well as embodying one of the reasons why Mrs. Shalev found life good for so very many decades. What seems hard to understand from the perspective of the treatment team and is altogether

225

unintelligible from the perspective of a rational, calculating self-asserter, may come to seem very reasonable indeed when seen in the context of that story. For example, while Mrs. Shalev is not an observant Jew, the variety of Judaism practiced in her community during her girlhood in the 1920s and 30s was hardly likely to be Reform. She comes out of a tradition that places a special value on life as a gift from God, a tradition that may be seen as vitalist. This tradition may well form an important part of the backdrop against which Mrs. Shalev's life can best be understood—her meticulousness about her medical care, for instance.

Further, if Ms. Putnam heard her mother say "Pain, schmain" once when she herself was growing up, she must have heard it a thousand times. For Mrs. Shalev—as indeed for all of us—pain is "necessary" or "unnecessary" only with respect to what hinges on accepting or rejecting it. If Mrs. Shalev did indeed value life and prize relationship as her daughter suggests, then there may in fact be nothing "unnecessary" about the pain she is experiencing.

So, while Mrs. Shalev is without doubt a vulnerable adult, it is, to say the least, very unclear what care would be most appropriate for her. Is it from pain and "indignity" that she needs to be protected, or is it death and the end of relationship that are her primary enemies? If the staff can remove themselves from the imaginary story of the reasonable person buried within their patient, and look to her daughter as a source of a richer story in which pain and death have a more particular meaning, some of this unclarity could possibly be resolved. Certainly, the "strategic ethics" to which the treatment team wants to turn—namely, to good ideas for getting shut of Ms. Putnam—would be replaced by a real ethical discussion, in which the prespectives of everyone involved in Mrs. Shalev's care could emerge. This would provide some space in which the possibilities of consensus or compromise could be explored. For instance, perhaps Ms. Putnam's views about the danger of analgesics for her mother are unrealistic, and a mutually acceptable pain control regimen could be achieved. Perhaps the timing of Ms. Putnam's visits to her mother could be adjusted to coincide with Mrs. Shalev's most lucid periods—periods in which dressing changes and other painful manipulations were not occuring.

Of course, as things happen, this strategy might not work out. There might actually be "unresolved issues" between Mrs. Shalev and her daughter that are being played out in a sort of perverse psychodrama with the health care team as unwilling participants. But Mrs. Shalev's caretakers might be in a much better position to make this judgment if, instead of being held captive by the "reasonable person" picture of their patient, they were more accepting of Ms. Putnam's account of her mother's life—if they allowed her to participate in the activity of maintaining her mother's selfhood even in the face of debilitating illness and a foreign, medical culture. If no compromise can be worked out, perhaps there is greater reason to suspect Ms. Putnam's motives and understandings. But the health care team, too, must be willing to compromise, or we will be suspicious of *their* motives and understandings. As difficult as this may be to accept, if the team is not willing to embrace a treatment regimen that may involve more interventions and more pain than they themselves would regard as appropriate, then they may well be imposing their own schemes of self-gratification on the defenseless body of someone whose good must be understood differently.

To treat Mrs. Shalev appropriately means to treat her as Mrs. Shalev, not as someone else. While the kinds of moral theories that guide contemporary health care workers would no doubt agree with this, the models that guide their imaginations pull against their own conviction. The model of the reasonable person isn't invoked only as a last resort, a default option to be turned to when all other avenues into an understanding of the patient's life have been blocked off; in this case, Ms. Putnam was there, had been there through much of Mrs. Shalev's life, and had given the caregivers no reason to doubt her own competence or her affection for her mother. Besides, the model of personhood the staff has invoked is no neutral conception of the self, embodying all and only those values that the generic reasonable person would have. There's nothing inherently unreasonable in the desire to live and to stay in relationship with one's intimates, even if the cost of doing so is physical suffering. A perspective that hands pain a trump card is not neutral, but rather an expression of the animating values of the health care professions. The kind of discussion we envisaged Ms. Putnam and the team engaging in after they had dropped their suspicion of each other's bona fides is an attempt to search together for sharable ground, each helping the other to see the sources of their moral concerns.

227

In some ways, Mrs. Shalev's case is fairly easy to think through, armed with the perspectives advocated here. There will be—and indeed are—harder issues involved in coming to grips with the particularities of people in the distinct circles, both of culture and of family, from which they come. For instance, the belief in the emigrant Hmong community in Minneapolis is that the leading males in a family should make its medical decisions—including decisions concerning the reproductive health of the family's adult women. Should decisions about cesarean sections or abortion be made by husbands rather than by wives? Here we encounter not only a different way of structuring decisionmaking authority than currently passes muster in American medical culture, but one that uncomfortably reminds us of our own history of misogyny, a history we are trying to put behind us. Determining which set of human goods to respect and which to sacrifice, when such goods stand in direct conflict, is never easy, nor will a given set of priorities answer in every case and at every moment in time.

Clashes among goods are going to occur more and more frequently as the mainstream of American society attempts to acknowledge and honor the diversity that exists within the country, instead of ignoring difference or trying to assimilate it so that it will disappear. The most hopeful long-term possibility for mediating these clashes is to temper our commitment to the kind of illusory neutrality that threatens to turn people into ghosts, and to move toward a truer "fusion of horizons," to use a term popularized by the philosopher Charles Taylor.[3] That is not to say that we should abdicate our own standards in favor of other ways of living in the world, of valuing and deciding, but that we should make every effort of imagination and education to become attentive to the sources of meaning and motivation that other cultures have found good.

In hospitals, clinics, and nursing homes, and in the offices of practitioners, this fusing of horizons can only take place by allowing the space for patients and their intimates to bring their own resources of meaning and caring to bear on the task of understanding and responding to illness, trauma, and other medical problems. The first step is to create a medicine that recaptures what must have been an old insight—that medical interventions can harm families, can disrupt their important functions, and must be observed to avoid such untoward outcomes. But medicine can no longer afford merely to remind itself to behave well in other people's houses; it must determine how to be welcoming to families, to cooperate with rather than defang them. It must understand both why families are important and how to enlist that importance in service of patient care.

The problems that moved the Clinton Administration to put health care reform at the head of its domestic agenda did not vanish when its hopes for passing legislation did. Reform remains inevitable, and in facing its necessity, Americans may come to learn much about medicine and health care, and may adjust their attitudes toward these fields as well. Indeed, the most thoughtful commentators today insist that this must happen if the reform is to have any real chance of solving some of our endemic problems. What has been much less marked is the idea that the health care system must come to new understandings and new attitudes about Americans—in particular, new understandings about both the intimate and the social networks in which they are embedded. While there's no guarantee that health care reform will include this kind of moral reconfiguration, making medicine a more homely place is a good way to move toward it.

References

Chapter One: A Rivalry of Care

1. This story is a variant on Case #2, found in Tom Beauchamp and James Childress, *Principles of Biomedical Ethics*, 2d ed. (New York: Oxford University Press, 1983), p. 285.
2. The classic discussion of this theme is John Hardwig's "What about the Family?" *Hastings Center Report* 20, no. 2 (1990): 5–10.
3. The account of the history of American medicine that follows is based on that of Paul Starr, *The Social Transformation of American Medicine: The Rise of a Sovereign Profession and the Making of a Vast Industry* (New York: Basic, 1982).
4. The following account of the history of the family is based on that of Steven Mintz and Susan Kellogg, *Domestic Revolutions: A Social History of American Family Life* (New York: Free Press, 1988).
5. Magali Sarfatti Larson, *The Rise of Professionalism* (Berkeley and Los Angeles: University of California Press, 1977), p. 14.
6. David Hume, *Treatise of Human Nature*, ed. L. A. Selby-Bigge (Oxford: Oxford University Press, 1951), p. 415.
7. Jane Austen, *Pride and Prejudice*, ed. R. W. Chapman, 3d ed. (Oxford: Oxford University Press, 1932), p. 216.
8. Alexis de Tocqueville, *Democracy in America*, ed. Phillips Bradley (New York: Alfred Knopf, 1945), 1:315; 2:202–4.
9. William J. Goode, *The Family*, 2d ed. (Englewood Cliffs, N.J.: Prentice-Hall, 1982), p. 7.

231

10. Ronald L. Numbers, "Do-It-Yourself the Sectarian Way," in *Medicine Without Doctors*, ed. Guenter B. Risse, Ronald L. Numbers, and Judith Walzer Leavitt (New York: Science History Publications, 1977).

11. Quoted in Numbers, "Do-It-Yourself," p. 58.

12. Numbers, "Do-It-Yourself," pp. 62–67.

13. Quoted in Starr, *Social Transformation*, p. 69.

14. Starr, *Social Transformation*, p. 151.

15. Henry Hurd, "The Hospital as a Factor in Modern Society," *The Modern Hospital* 1 (September 1913): 33.

16. Quoted in Starr, *Social Transformation*, p. 134.

17. Edwin Shorter, *The Health Century* (New York: Doubleday, 1987), pp. 6–19.

18. John C. Burnham, "America's Golden Age: What Happened to It?" in *Sickness & Health in America*, ed. Judith Walzer Leavitt and Ronald L. Numbers (Madison: University of Wisconsin Press, 1985), pp. 248–58.

19. See Christopher Lasch, *Haven in a Heartless World: The Family Besieged* (New York: Basic Books, 1977), pp. 8–9.

20. Kellogg and Mintz, *Domestic Revolutions*, p. 116.

21. Robert Jay Lifton, *The Nazi Doctors: Medical Killing and the Psychology of Genocide* (New York: Basic Books, 1986), p. 22.

22. William Butler Yeats, "The Second Coming," in *The Collected Poems* (New York: Macmillan, 1956), pp. 184–85.

23. Starr, *Social Transformation of American Medicine*, p. 258.

24. Michael M. Davis, Jr., "The American Approach to Health Insurance," *Milbank Memorial Fund Quarterly* 12 (July 1934): 214–15.

25. Starr, *Social Transformation of American Medicine*, p. 271.

26. Burnham, "America's Golden Age," p. 249.

27. Patricia L. Kendall, "Medical Specialization: Trends and Contributing Factors," in *Psychosocial Aspects of Medical Training*, ed. R. H. Coombs and C. E. Vincent (Springfield, Ill.: C. C. Thomas, 1971).

28. Starr, *Social Transformation of American Medicine*, p. 384.

29. See the survey conducted by the Children's Defense Fund, as reported in the *Washington Post*, 22 May 1991.

30. See Philip Elmer-Devitt, "The Crucial Early Years," *Time*, 18 April 1994, which summarizes the Carnegie report. These statistics must be interpreted with caution, however. It is true that prenatal care in the U.S. is haphazard and inadequate, but it is also true that in this country the standard of care is to try to save the lives of very-low-birthweight babies who in other countries would be allowed to die and not counted among live births.

31. Starr, *Social Transformation of American Medicine*, p. 410.

32. Kellogg and Mintz, *Domestic Revolutions*, p. 162.

33. Quoted in Kellogg and Mintz, *Domestic Revolutions*, p. 181.

34. Carnegie Corporation report, in Elmer-Devitt, "Crucial Early Years."

35. National Center for Health Statistics, 1985 projections released in November 1991, in conversation, 12 December 1991.

36. The statistics in this paragraph are found in Susan Moller Okin, *Justice, Gender, and the Family* (New York: Basic Books, 1989); the quotation is from pp. 161–62.

37. See the Carnegie Corporation report, Elmer-Devitt, "The Crucial Early Years," and Okin, *Justice, Gender, and the Family*, p. 160.
38. Kellogg and Mintz, *Domestic Revolutions*, pp. 213, 217.
39. Kellogg and Mintz, *Domestic Revolutions*, pp. 242–43.
40. Caroline Wolf Harlow, *Female Victims of Violent Crime* (Washington, D.C.: U.S. Department of Justice, Bureau of Justice Statistics, 1991), pp. 1–7.
41. See "Women and Violence: Hearings before the Senate Committee on the Judiciary," 101st Cong., 2d Sess. 117 (1990), testimony of Angela Browne, Ph.D.
42. Margaret Crosbie-Burnett, "Impact of Joint versus Sole Custody and Quality of Co-parental Relationship on Adjustment of Adolescents in Remarried Families," *Behavioral Sciences and the Law* 9 (Autumn 1991): 439–49.
43. This story is a retelling from Janet Haas, Arthur Caplan, and Daniel Callahan, eds., *Case Studies in Ethics and Medical Rehabilitation* (Briarcliff Manor, N.Y.: The Hastings Center, 1988), pp. 1–2.
44. This story is taken from Pete Busalacchi, "How Can They?" *Hastings Center Report* 20, no. 5 (1990): 6–7; Brian McCormick, "Case Looks at Parental Rights in Medical Decisions," *American Medical News,* 21 October 1991; "Comatose Woman, Focus of Court Battles, Dies," *New York Times,* 8 March 1993.

Chapter Two: Why Families Matter

1. William J. Goode, *The Family*, 2d ed. (Englewood Cliffs, N.J.: Prentice-Hall, 1982), p. 171.
2. National Center for Health Statistics, 1985 projections released in November 1991.
3. See, for example, Shulamith Firestone, *The Dialectic of Sex* (New York: William Morrow, 1970); Hugh LaFollette, "Licensing Parents," *Philosophy and Public Affairs* 9 (Winter 1980): 182–97.
4. John Rawls, *A Theory of Justice* (Cambridge: Harvard University Press, 1971), p. 74. In fairness to Rawls, he does argue that, in the context of his overall theory, the "urgency" to achieve perfect equality of opportunity is "reduced" (p. 301).
5. See, for example, President George Bush's campaign speech, reported in the *New York Times,* 10 March 1992.
6. David Hume, *Enquiries Concerning Human Understanding and Concerning the Principles of Morals* (Oxford: Oxford University Press, 3rd edition, 1975), p. 185.
7. Michael Sandel, *Liberalism and the Limits of Justice* (Cambridge: Cambridge University Press, 1982), pp. 33–34.
8. Fred Rosner, "A Breakdown in the Family Unit," *Journal of Clinical Ethics* 2, no. 3 (1991): 149.
9. For the distinction between the family as household and the family in the abstract, see Patricia Smith, "Family Responsibility and the Nature of Obligation," in *Kindred Matters: Rethinking the Philosophy of the Family,* ed. Diana Tietjens Meyers, Kenneth Kipnis, and Cornelius F. Murphy, Jr. (Ithaca: Cornell University Press, 1993), p. 47.
10. Sara Ruddick, *Maternal Thinking: Toward a Politics of Peace* (Boston: Beacon Press, 1989). The tasks of maternal work are listed on p. 17. It should be noted that birthgiving is not regarded as a part of maternal work proper; for this reason, Ruddick argues, maternal work is in principle open to either gender.

11. Goode, *The Family*, p. 6.
12. Salvador Minuchin, *Families and Family Therapy* (Cambridge, Mass.: Harvard University Press, 1974), pp. 47–48.
13. See data from the Carnegie report in Philip Elmer-Dewitt, "The Crucial Early Years," *Time*, 18 April 1994.
14. E. Bijur et al., "Parental Alcohol Use, Problem Drinking, and Children's Injuries," *JAMA* 267, no. 23 (1992): 3166–71.
15. Teri Randall, "Adolescents May Experience Home, School Abuse; Their Future Draws Researchers' Concern," *JAMA* 267, no. 23 (1992): 3127–28, 3131, at 3127.
16. William F. May, "The Molested," in *The Patient's Ordeal* (Bloomington: Indiana University Press, 1991).
17. May, "The Molested," as reprinted in the *Hastings Center Report* 21, no. 3 (1991): 9–17, at 11.
18. Howard Brody, *The Healer's Power* (New Haven, Conn.: Yale University Press, 1992), p. 43.
19. Laura M. Purdy, *In Their Best Interest? The Case against Equal Rights for Children* (Ithaca: Cornell University Press, 1992), p. 64.
20. Vance Packard, *Our Endangered Children* (Boston: Little, Brown, 1983), p. 8, quoted in Purdy, *In Their Best Interest?*
21. Margaret Urban Walker, "Moral Particularity," *Metaphilosophy* 18, nos. 3, 4 (1987): 171–85.
22. John Rawls, *A Theory of Justice*, pp. 62, 178. Acknowledging the significance of self-respect raises a problem for any position which, like Rawls's, flirts with the idea that a society purged of families might be morally more admirable than traditional societies: how, outside of small-scale social structures in which individuals can be known and prized in a way that is highly attuned to their particular characteristics, can the foundation for self-esteem be laid?
23. For a powerful and vivid explanation of the moral significance of this fact, see Bernard Williams, "Persons, Character and Morality," in *Moral Luck* (Cambridge: Cambridge University Press, 1981), pp. 1–19.
24. Eric J. Cassell, "Recognizing Suffering," *Hastings Center Report* 21, no. 3 (1991): 24–31, at 25.
25. We are indebted to Joseph J. Fins, M.D., an assistant professor of medicine at New York Hospital-Cornell Medical Center, for guiding the Pisanis through the hospital for us.
26. Redford B. Williams et al., "Prognostic Importance of Social and Economic Resources among Medically Treated Patients with Angiographically Documented Coronary Artery Disease," *JAMA* 267, no. 4 (1992): 520–24; Blair Justice, *Who Gets Sick: How Beliefs, Moods, and Thoughts Affect Your Health* (Los Angeles: Jeremy P. Tarcher, 1988); Jane Brody, "Maintaining Friendships for the Sake of Your Health," *New York Times*, 5 February 1992. For what happens after Mr. Pisani leaves the hospital, see Wayne M. Sotile, *Heart Illness and Intimacy: How Caring Relationships Aid Recovery* (Baltimore: Johns Hopkins University Press, 1992).
27. Nancy M. P. King, "Transparency in Neonatal Intensive Care," *Hastings Center Report* 22, no. 3 (1992): 18–25.
28. Perri Klass, *Other Women's Children* (New York: Random House, 1990), p. 147.
29. Thanks to Ellen McAvoy for this story.

Chapter Three: An Ethics for Families

1. John Hardwig, "In Search of an Ethics of Personal Relationships," in *Person to Person*, ed. George Graham and Hugh LaFolette (Philadelphia: Temple University Press, 1989), p. 63.

2. Martha Minow, *Making All the Difference: Inclusion, Exclusion, and American Law* (Ithaca and London: Cornell University Press, 1990).

3. For an interesting thought-experiment along these lines see Thomas Donaldson, "Morally Privileged Relationships," in *Kindred Matters: Rethinking the Philosophy of the Family*, ed. Diana Tietjens Meyers, Kenneth Kipnis, and Cornelius F. Murphy, Jr. (Ithaca: Cornell University Press, 1993), pp. 21–40.

4. See, for example, the reservations voiced in James Lindemann Nelson, "Parenthood and Partialism," *Journal of Social Philosophy* 21, no. 1 (Spring 1990): 107–18.

5. Margaret Urban Walker, "Moral Particularity," *Metaphilosophy* 18, no. 3/4 (1987): 171–85.

6. A phrase introduced into the literature by Thomas Nagel. See his *The View from Nowhere* (Oxford: Oxford University Press, 1986).

7. Bernard Williams, "Persons, Character and Morality," in *Moral Luck* (New York: Cambridge University Press), pp. 1–19.

8. These issues have been sensitively probed in a series of publications by E. Haavi Morreim. See in particular her *Balancing Act: The New Medical Ethics of Medicine's New Economics* (Dordrecht, the Netherlands: Kluwer, 1991).

9. See Rebecca Dresser, "Wanted: Single, White Male for Medical Research," *Hastings Center Report* 22, no. 1 (1992): 24–29; and Nancy Jecker, "Can an Employer-Based Health Insurance System Be Just?" *Journal of Health Politics, Policy and Law* 18, no. 3 (1993).

10. The classic texts in contemporary bioethics include Tom Beauchamp and James F. Childress, *Principles of Biomedical Ethics* (New York: Oxford University Press, 1994), now in its fourth edition; an excellent anthology surveying the field is John Arras and Bonnie Steinbock, eds., *Ethical Issues in Modern Medicine* (Mountain View, Cal.: Mayfield Publishing, 1995), in its fourth edition.

11. See Thomas Nagel's *Equality and Partiality* (New York: Oxford University Press, 1991).

12. Williams, "Persons, Character and Morality," p. 18.

13. For one example of the assumption that obligation is based on consent, see Eike-Henner W. Kluge, "Designated Organ Donation: Private Choice in Social Context," *Hastings Center Report* 19, no. 5 (1989): 10–16. For another example (in the form of a claim that specific rights arise only from the voluntary acts of others), see Laurence D. Houlgate, "Ethical Theory and the Family," in *Kindred Matters*.

14. A wealth of data on domestic violence and the comparative severity of its effects were collected in *JAMA* 267, no. 23 (17 June 1992).

15. See Williams, "Persons, Character and Morality," and John Rawls, *A Theory of Justice* (Cambridge, Mass.: The Belknap Press of Harvard University Press, 1972).

16. Henry Sidgwick, *The Methods of Ethics*, 7th ed. (Chicago: The University of Chicago Press, 1907), p. 243.

17. Jerome Kagan, *The Nature of the Child* (New York: Basic Books, 1984), pp 119–20.

18. See also William Damon, *The Moral Child: Nurturing Children's Natural Moral Growth* (New York: Free Press, 1988).
19. Jiao, G. Ji, and Q. Jing, "Comparative Study of Behavioral Qualities of Only Children and Sibling Children," *Child Development* 57 (1986): 357–61.
20. For a wise and rich account of conscience see Martin Benjamin's entry s.v. "Conscience," *Encyclopedia of Bioethics,* 2d ed. (New York: Macmillan, 1995).
21. Larry Blum, *Friendship, Altruism and Morality* (Boston: Routledge & Kegan Paul, 1980).

Chapter Four: Medical Decisionmaking

1. N.Y. 128, 105 N.E. 93 (1914). See the discussion in Ruth R. Faden and Tom L. Beauchamp, *A History and Theory of Informed Consent* (Oxford: Oxford University Press, 1986), p. 123.
2. See the President's Commission for the Study of Ethical Problems in Medicine and Biomedical and Behavioral Research, *Making Health Care Decisions* (Washington, D.C.: U.S. Government Printing Office, 1982); Tom L. Beauchamp and James F. Childress, *Principles of Biomedical Ethics,* 4th ed. (New York: Oxford University Press, 1994).
3. A particularly clear-headed and readable treatment of this topic is Howard Brody's *Healer's Power* (New Haven: Yale University Press, 1992).
4. We're pleased to note that in the fourth edition of this influential text (1994) the special moral character of the family is more explicitly acknowledged.
5. Allen E. Buchanan and Dan W. Brock, *Deciding for Others: The Ethics of Surrogate Decision Making* (Cambridge: Cambridge University Press), pp. 136–37, 143.
6. In re Quinlan, 70 NJ 10 (1976).
7. In re Jobes, 108 NJ 394 (1987).
8. In re Jobes.
9. For a closer look at the data, most of it concerning elderly patients and their families, see R. F. Uhlmann, R. A. Pearlman, and K. C. Cain, "Physicians' and Spouses' Predictions of Elderly Patients' Resuscitation Preferences," *Journal of Gerontology* 43, supplement (1988): M115–M121; A. B. Seckler, D. E. Meier, M. Mulvihill, B. E. Canmer Paris, "Substituted Judgment: How Accurate Are Proxy Predictions?" *Annals of Internal Medicine* 115 (1991): 92–98; N. R. Zweibel and C. K. Cassel, "Treatment Choices at the End of Life: A Comparison of Decisions by Older Patients and Their Physician-Selected Proxies," *Gerontologist* 29 (1989): 615–21; Tom Tomlinson, K. Howe, M. Notman, D. Rossmiller, "An Empirical Study of Proxy Consent for Elderly Persons," *Gerontologist* 30 (1990): 54–61; J. G. Ouslander, A. J. Tymchuk, and B. Rahbar, "Health Care Decisions among Elderly Long-Term Care Residents and Their Potential Proxies," *Archives of Internal Medicine* 149 (1989): 1367–72.
10. Patricia D. White, in conversation and in her article, "Appointing a Proxy under the Best of Circumstances," *Utah Law Review* 1992, no. 3 (1992): 851.
11. See Buchanan and Brock, *Deciding for Others;* President's Commission for the Study of Ethical Problems in Medicine and Biomedical and Behavioral Research, *Deciding to Forego Life-Sustaining Treatment* (Washington, D.C.: U.S. Government Printing Office, 1983), ch. 4; *In re Jobes,* 108 N.J. 394 (1987); George J. Annas, "The Health Care Proxy and the Living Will," *NEJM* 324 (1991): 1210–13; *Life-Sustaining*

Treatment: Making Decisions and Appointing a Health Care Agent (New York: New York State Task Force on Life and the Law, 1987) ch. 4; "Practicing the PSDA," Special Supplement, *Hastings Center Report* 21, no. 5 (1991).

12. This description of best interests, adapted from Buchanan and Brock, *Deciding for Others*, p. 94, is fairly standard.

13. Linda Emanuel, "PSDA in the Clinic," in "Practicing the PSDA," Special Supplement, *Hastings Center Report* 21, no. 5 (1991): S6–S7.

14. Rebecca Dresser, "Missing Persons: Legal Perceptions of Incompetent Patients," *Rutgers Law Review* 46, no. 2 (1994): 609–719.

15. See Ezekiel J. Emanuel and Linda L. Emanuel, "Proxy Decision Making for Incompetent Patients: An Ethical and Empirical Analysis," *JAMA* 267, no. 15 (1992): 2067–71; also Ezekiel Emanuel, *The Ends of Human Life: Medical Ethics in a Liberal Polity* (Cambridge, Mass.: Harvard University Press, 1991); and Linda L. Emanuel and Ezekiel J. Emanuel, "Decisions at the End of Life: Guided by Communities of Patients," *Hastings Center Report* 23, no. 5 (1993): 6–14.

16. Emanuel and Emanuel, "Proxy Decision Making," p. 2071.

17. Emanuel and Emanuel, "Proxy Decision Making," p. 2071.

18. Emanuel and Emanuel, "Proxy Decision Making."

19. See James Lindemann Nelson and Hilde Lindemann Nelson, "Guided by Intimates," *Hastings Center Report* 23, no. 5 (1993): 14–15.

20. Joanne Lynn, "Why I Don't Have a Living Will," *Law, Medicine, and Health Care* 19 (1991): 101–4.

21. Lisa Belkin, "In Right-to-Die Fight, Court Finds Family Liable for Care," *New York Times* metro section, 24 September 1992.

22. The break is not gender-neutral. Susan Muller Okin, quoting Lenore Weitzman's *The Divorce Revolution*, reports that after divorce, ninety percent of dependent children live with their mothers. If a child's chronic illness or disability has put intolerable pressure on a fragile marriage, the father is likely to leave while the mother stays and cares for the child. See Okin, *Justice, Gender, and the Family* (New York: Basic Books, 1989), pp. 160–62. Tamar Lewin, "Rise in Single Parenting Is Reshaping U.S.," *New York Times*, 5 October 1992, reports that only 3.8 percent of white single-parent households are headed by fathers, while for black and hispanic households the figure is 4.5 percent.

23. Tamar Lewin, "Disabled Woman's Lesbian Partner Is Granted Right to Be Her Guardian," *New York Times*, 18 December 1991.

24. For a fictional account of how a wife creates such an atmosphere when she comes to understand that the man she has married possesses a vicious character, see Anthony Trollope's *The Prime Minister*. In that novel, Elizabeth Wharton Lopez builds her own married life around the reality of Ferdinand Lopez's badness.

25. See Benjamin Freedman, Abraham Fuks, and Charles Weijer, "*In Loco Parentis*: Minimal Risk as an Ethical Threshold for Research upon Children," *Hastings Center Report* 23, no. 2 (1993): 13–19.

26. See Michael Lipson, "What Do You Say to a Child with AIDS?" *Hastings Center Report* 23, no. 2 (1993): 6–12.

27. Office of Technology Assessment, *Adolescent Health*, vol. 1, *Summary and Policy Options*, OTA–H–468 (Washington, D.C.: U.S. Government Printing Office, April 1991).

28. Alison M. Jaggar, "Abortion and a Woman's Right to Decide," in *Living with Contradictions: Controversies in Feminist Social Ethics*, ed. Alison M. Jaggar (Boulder: Westview Press, 1994), p. 282.

29. Margaret Urban Walker, "Moral Particularity," *Metaphilosophy* 18, no. 3/4 (1987): 171–85.

30. The idea for this story came from John Hardwig, in a talk he gave at The Hastings Center in March 1991.

31. J. Stein and C. W. G. Redman, "Maternal-Fetal Conflict: A Definition," *Medico-Legal Journal* 58, pt. 4 (1990): 230–35.

32. John Hardwig, "What about the Family?" *Hastings Center Report* 20, no. 2 (1990): 5–10.

33. These themes are discussed further in James Lindemann Nelson, "Taking Families Seriously," *Hastings Center Report* 22, no. 4 (1992): 6–12.

34. Howard Brody, "Transparency: Informed Consent in Primary Care," *Hastings Center Report* 19, no. 5 (1989): 5–9.

35. For a lucid and careful exposition of this idea, see Margaret Urban Walker, "Keeping Moral Space Open: New Images of Ethics Consulting," *Hastings Center Report*, 23, no. 2 (1993): 33–40.

Chapter Five: When I'm Sixty-Four

1. Daniel Callahan, *Setting Limits: Medical Goals in an Aging Society* (New York: Simon and Schuster, 1987), p. 21; also Elaine M. Brody, *Women in the Middle: Their Parent-Care Years* (New York: Springer, 1990), pp. 6–9, 13.

2. See Daniel Callahan, *The Troubled Dream of Life: Living with Mortality* (New York: Simon and Schuster, 1993).

3. Callahan, *Setting Limits*, p. 19.

4. Rosenmayhr and E. Kockeis, "Propositions for a Sociological Theory of Aging and the Family," *International Social Science Journal* 15 (1963): 410–26.

5. Pillimer and D. Finkelhor, "The Prevalence of Elder Abuse: A Random Sample Survey," *Gerontologist* 28 (1988): 51–57.

6. Callahan, *Setting Limits*, p. 44. See also the Summer 1992 issue of *Generations: Journal of the American Society on Aging*, which is devoted to a multicultural look at families and aging. For a nice précis of the myths of aging see Brody, *Women in the Middle*, p. 19.

7. Brody, *Women in the Middle*, pp. 80–82.

8. Nancy Guberman, "The Family, Women and Caring: Who Cares for the Carers?" *Resources for Feminist Research* 17, no. 2 (1988): 37–40, at 38.

9. For Aristotle's views, see *Nicomachean Ethics*, 1163b: "This is why it would not seem open to a man to disown his father (though a father may disown a son); being in debt, he should repay, but there is nothing by doing which a son will have done the equivalent of what he has received, so that he is always in debt." For Aquinas, see *Summa Theologica*, question 101, article 1, in which he asserts that since our parents are, next to God, the "closest sources of our existence and development," we owe them respect, reverence, and services.

10. Sir William Blackstone, *Commentaries on The Laws of England*, vol. 1 (Philadelphia: J. B. Lippincott and Co. 1856), bk. 1, ch. 16, section 1, quoted in

Jeffrey Blustein, *Parents and Children: The Ethics of the Family* (New York: Oxford, 1982), p. 181.

11. Christina Hoff Sommers, "Filial Morality," *Journal of Philosophy* 83, no. 8 (1986): 439–56, at 446–47.

12. Jane English, "What Do Grown Children Owe Their Parents?" in *Having Children: Philosophical and Legal Reflections on Parenthood*, ed. Onora O'Neill and William Ruddick (New York: Oxford University Press, 1979), pp. 351–56.

13. Mark R. Wicclair, "Caring for Frail Elderly Parents: Past Parental Sacrifices and the Obligations of Adult Children," *Social Theory and Practice* 16, no. 2 (1990): 163–89; see also his *Ethics and the Elderly* (New York: Oxford University Press, 1993), ch. 6.

14. Joel Feinberg, "Duties, Rights, and Claims," *American Philosophical Quarterly* 3 (1966): 139.

15. Blustein, *Parents and Children*, p. 183.

16. Colin Turnbull, *The Mountain People* (1974; New York: Peter Smith, 1988).

17. James Joyce, *A Portrait of the Artist as a Young Man* (New York: Viking, 1964), p. 7.

18. Christine M. Korsgaard, "Morality as Freedom," in *Kant's Practical Philosophy Reconsidered*, ed. Yirmiahu, Yovel (Dordrecht, The Netherlands: Kluwer, 1989), pp. 23–48, at 45.

19. For a very helpful discussion of this point, see Annette C. Baier, "The Need for More than Justice," in *Science, Morality, and Feminist Theory*, ed. Marsha Hanen and Kai Nielsen, special supplement, *Canadian Journal of Philosophy* 13 (1987).

20. This story is told with apologies to Margaret Urban Walker, "Moral Particularity," *Metaphilosophy* 18, nos. 3 & 4 (1987): 171–84, at 171.

21. Adapted from Brody, *Women in the Middle*, pp. 157–58.

22. Charles Taylor, *The Ethics of Authenticity* (Cambridge, Mass: Harvard University Press, 1991).

23. Norman Daniels, *Am I My Parents' Keeper? An Essay on Justice between the Young and the Old* (New York: Oxford University Press, 1988), pp. 69–82.

24. We are indebted for this image, as for much of the thinking in this chapter, to Daniel Callahan.

25. Callahan, *Setting Limits*, pp. 31–32.

26. Jim Lubitz, of the Health Care Financing Administration, personal communication, 22 June 1992.

27. Pamphlet, "A Profile of Older Americans: 1992," produced by the American Association of Retired Persons and the Administration on Aging, U.S. Department of Health and Human Services.

28. "Cost of Heart Revival Put at $150,000 per Survivor," *New York Times*, 21 March 1993.

29. This account is adapted from Ronald E. Cranford, "Helga Wanglie's Ventilator," *Hastings Center Report* 21, no. 4 (1991): 23–24.

30. Nancy M. P. King, "Transparency in Neonatal Intensive Care," *Hastings Center Report* 22, no. 3 (1992): 20ff.

31. For a discussion of the role of social values in futility decisions, see Daniel Callahan, "Medical Futility, Medical Necessity: The Problem-Without-A-Name," *Hastings Center Report* 21, no. 4 (1991): 30–35.

32. This case is adapted from Case Study: "Letting Her Go," *Hastings Center Report* 22, no. 6 (1992): 26.

33. Bruce Jennings, "Last Rights: Dying and the Limits of Self-Sovereignty," *In Depth* 2, no. 3 (1992): 103–18.

34. Nancy Neveloff Dubler and David Nimmons, *Ethics on Call: A Medical Ethicist Shows How to Take Charge of Life and Death Choices* (New York: Harmony Books, 1992).

35. For a survey of the major arguments in this debate, see Joseph Jack Fins and Matthew D. Bacchetta, "The Physician-Assisted Suicide and Euthanasia Debate: An Annotated Bibliography of Representative Articles," *Journal of Clinical Ethics* 5, no. 4 (1994).

Chapter Six: When Medicine Makes Babies

1. This figure, the most recent one available from the federal government, is from the Office of Technology Assessment, *Infertility: Medical and Social Choices* (Washington, D.C.: United States Printing Office, 1988).

2. The figures are taken from Sharon Elizabeth Rush, "Breaking with Tradition: Surrogacy and Gay Fathers," in *Kindred Matters: Rethinking the Philosophy of the Family*, ed. Diana Tietjens Meyers, Kenneth Kipnis, and Cornelius F. Murphy, Jr. (Ithaca: Cornell University Press, 1993), p. 121.

3. For an interesting discussion of responses to infertility, see Antonia Abbey, Frank M. Andrews and L. Jill Halman, "Gender's Role in Responses to Infertility," *Psychology of Women Quarterly* 15 (1991): 295–316.

4. This account was drawn from "When One Body Can Save Another," *Time*, 17 June 1991, p. 54; and from "One Year after Ayala Transplant, a Wedding," *American Medical News*, 6–13 July 1992, p. 42.

5. B. D. Colen, "The Price of Life," *New York Newsday*, 11 March 1990.

6. For arguments that parental obligations come from voluntary undertakings see Onora O'Neill, "Begetting, Bearing, and Rearing," in *Having Children: Philosophical and Legal Reflections*, ed. Onora O'Neill and William Ruddick (New York: Oxford University Press, 1979).

7. Sara Ruddick, in conversation, October 1987.

8. In conversation, November 1991.

9. Ethics Committee of the American Fertility Society, "Ethical Considerations of the New Reproductive Technologies," supplement 2, *Fertility and Sterility* 53, no. 6 (June 1990): 418.

10. Office of Technology Assessment, *Infertility*, attributes this estimate to Bill Handel, who runs the largest contract pregnancy brokerage in California. Because the 1988 OTA report is the most recent white paper on the subject issued by the government, the "four thousand" figure keeps being cited; it crops up in the April 1992 New York State Department of Health's "The Business of Surrogate Parenting," for example.

11. The cost of IVF is taken from the Office of Technology Assessment, *Infertility*. Other figures are from New York State Department of Health, "The Business of Surrogate Parenting," whose 1992 figures are quite similar to those the OTA used in 1988.

12. The age of the woman whose egg is used is a factor, too. If she is young enough, the success rate can go as high as forty percent. American Fertility Society, "Ethical Considerations," p. 39S, cites the National IVF–ET Registry of the United

States' sixteen percent figure. On p. 37S we read, "Currently, the success rates vary but have been reported to be up to 25% per cycle of treatment."

13. New York State Department of Health, "Business of Surrogate Parenting," p. 7.

14. Janice Raymond, "Reproductive Gifts and Gift Giving: The Altruistic Woman," *Hastings Center Report* 20, no. 6 (1990): 7–11.

15. *Johnson v. Calvert,* Cal. Super. Ct., Orange Co., Dept 11, No. X633190 (22 Oct. 1990).

16. *Anna J. v. Mark C.,* 286 Cal. Rptr. 369 (Ct. App., 4th Dist, 1991).

17. See the *Washington Post,* 26 November 1991.

18. See Medical Research International and Society for Assisted Reproduction of The American Fertility Society, "In Vitro Fertilization-Embryo Transfer (IVF-ET) in the United States: 1990 Results from the IVF–ET Registry," *Fertility and Sterility* 57 (1992): 15–24.

19. Ellen Moskowitz, "Blinded by Principle: The Tennessee Supreme Court's Contract Rule on Frozen Human Embryos" (Hastings Center, Briarcliff Manor, N.Y., 1992), unpublished manuscript.

20. See Kathleen Nolan, "*Genug ist Genug:* A Fetus Is Not a Kidney," *Hastings Center Report* 18, no. 6 (1988): 13–19.

21. Barbara Katz Rothman, *The Tentative Pregnancy: Prenatal Diagnosis and the Future of Motherhood* (New York: Viking, 1986), pp. 250–51.

22. These issues are examined in considerable depth in Derek Parfit, *Reasons and Persons* (New York: Oxford University Press, 1984), part 4.

23. See, among many other arguments, William Ruddick, "Are Fetuses Becoming Children?" in *Biomedical Ethics and Fetal Therapy,* ed. Carl Numrod and Glenn Griener (Calgary: Wilfrid Laurier University Press, 1988); see also his "When Does Childhood Begin?" in *Children, Parents, and Politics,* ed. Geoffrey Scarre (Cambridge: Cambridge University Press, 1989).

24. Robert Frost, "The Death of the Hired Man."

25. See Hilde Lindemann Nelson, "The Architect and the Bee: Some Reflections on Postmortem Pregnancy," *Bioethics* 8, no. 3 (1994): 247–67.

Chapter Seven: With Medicine and Justice for All

1. A recent study conducted at the University of Pennsylvania reported that half the children surveyed five years after divorce had not heard from their fathers for at least a year (Dirk Johnson, "More and More, Single Parent Is Dad," *New York Times,* 31 August 1993).

2. Preliminary results of the Global Utilization of Streptokinase & t-PA for Occluded Coronary Arteries trial (GUSTO) indicate that "myocardial infarction patients who received a front-loaded dose of the genetically engineered tissue plasminogen activator (t-PA) had a 14% lower mortality rate than those who received a steady infusion of streptokinase." See the report in *Medical World News* for May 1993, p. 13. The quote attributed to Dr. Schliermacher is actually from William Ganz, a cardiologist at the University of California at Los Angeles, reported in David Brown and Sally Squires, "Costly Drug Called Best Choice After Heart Attack," *Washington Post,* 1 May 1993. A study published in three consecutive issues of the *British Medical Journal* in January 1994 suggests that aspirin, at one cent a tablet, is just as effective a clot-destroyer as t-PA. It will be interesting to see what cardiologists make of this study.

3. See, for example, Rodney Peffer, *Marxism, Morality and Social Justice* (Princeton: Princeton University Press, 1989).

4. Notoriously, Robert Nozick, *Anarchy, State and Utopia* (New York: Basic Books, 1974).

5. For details of the most recent six-organ transplant, see Paul Menzel, "Rescuing Lives: Can't We Count?" *Hastings Center Report* 24, no. 1 (1994): 22–23.

6. John Rawls, *A Theory of Justice* (Cambridge, Mass.: Harvard University Press, 1971), p. 3.

7. James Rachels, "Morality, Parents and Children," in George Graham and Hugh LaFollette, *Person to Person* (Philadelphia: Temple University Press, 1989).

8. This may be because most people don't have gunshot wounds, or aren't making credible threats against others, or aren't HIV infected when they come to the doctor; those who fall into these categories may have other ideas about the matter.

9. Michael Walzer, *Spheres of Justice: A Defense of Pluralism and Equality* (New York: Basic Books, 1983), p. 7.

10. See, for instance, William Galston, "Review of Michael Walzer, *Spheres of Justice,*" *Ethics* 94, no. 2 (1984): 329–33.

11. See, for instance, the discussion in H. Hansmann, "The Economics and Ethics of Markets for Human Organs," *Journal of Health Politics, Policy and Law* 14, no. 1 (1989): 74.

12. See Susan Moller Okin's discussion of Barbara R. Bergmann's *The Economic Emergence of Women* (New York: Basic Books, 1986) in Okin, *Justice, Gender, and the Family* (New York: Basic Books, 1989), ch. 7.

13. See Richard Arneson, "Feminism and Family Justice," presented at the Central Division meetings of the American Philosophical Association, April 1993.

14. In "National Health Expenditures Projected through 2030," *Health Care Finance Review* 14, no. 1 (1992), Burner, Waldo and McKusick estimated that 1993 health care costs in the U.S. would amount to $3,380 per citizen—a total of over $900 billion. The trillion-dollar barrier was broken by 1994.

15. Council on Ethical and Judicial Affairs, "Gender Discrimination in the Medical Profession," *Women's Health Issues* 4, no. 1 (1994): 1–11.

16. See Rebecca Dresser, "Wanted: Single, White Male for Medical Research," *Hastings Center Report* 22, no. 1 (1992): 24–29.

17. Okin, *Justice, Gender and the Family*, p. 153.

18. Okin, *Justice, Gender and the Family*, pp. 180–83.

19. Okin, *Justice, Gender, and the Family*, pp. 124, 122. For a useful discussion of Okin's liberalizing of the family, see Will Kymlicka, "Rethinking the Family," *Philosophy and Public Affairs* 20, no. 1 (1991): 77–97.

20. Iris Marion Young, *Justice and the Politics of Difference* (Princeton: Princeton University Press, 1990). Young's particular emphasis is on the power differential within interpersonal relationships, but we are not focusing exclusively on power.

21. Richard Aronson, "Feminism and Family Justice."

22. Jane Austen, *Mansfield Park*, 3d ed. (Oxford: Oxford University Press, 1934), pp. 383, 392.

23. Inspired by a case discussed in *Bioethics: Readings and Cases*, ed. Baruch Brody and H. Tristram Englehardt, Jr. (New Jersey: Prentice-Hall, 1978) pp. 337–38.

24. Howard Brody, *The Healer's Power* (New Haven: Yale University Press, 1992), p. 186.

25. Brody, *The Healer's Power*, p. 190.
26. Adapted from "Please Don't Tell," *Hastings Center Report* 21, no. 6 (991): 39.
27. Marcia Angell, Commentary on "Please Don't Tell," p. 40.
28. See James Lindemann Nelson, *The Rights and Responsibilities of Potential Organ Donors: A Communitarian Approach* (Washington, D.C.: Communitarian Network, 1992).
29. See James Lindemann Nelson, "Families and Futility," *Journal of the American Geriatrics Society* 42, no. 8 (1994): 879–82.

Coda: Medicine, Families, and Other Sources of Identity

1. This analysis has been inspired by the work of Elizabeth V. Spelman, in particular, by her *Inessential Woman: Problems of Exclusion in Feminst Thought* (Boston: Beacon Press, 1988).
2. This case was drawn from material provided by Gay Moldow.
3. See Charles Taylor, *The Ethics of Authenticity* (Cambridge, Mass.: Harvard University Press, 1991). Taylor derives the idea from the German philosopher Hans-George Gadamer.

Index

Abortion: and feminism, 105-6; and genetic screening, 173-79; as alternative to adoption, 160; "Dr. Hunter's Dilemma," 103; "One Down Syndrome Too Many," 173-75; prohibition of, 16; teenage, 103-6

Abuse: fear of familial, 115-17; of elderly, 121; of intimates, 37-38, 70; of patient, 225; of women, 24-25

Aging: and families, 119-54, 193; and resource allocation, 202-3; ethics of caring for, 125-33; of society, 119; meaning of, 139-40; myths of, 121-22; setting limits on care for, 139-47

Aquinas, Saint Thomas, 126

Aristotle, 81, 126, 128

Aronson, Richard, 198

Austen, Jane, 198-99

Autonomy: "Caring for Tony," 26-28; of patient, 56, 117, 205; in medical ethics, 61-62; limits on, 151; "With His Boots On," 149-51

Ayala, Anissa, 157

Ayala, Marissa, 157

Ayala, Mary and Abe, 157

"Baby M": court case, 166, 167

Beneficence: as guide to decision-making, 83; in doctor-patient relationship, 206-9; in medical ethics, 61-62

Bentham, Jeremy, 58

Beauchamp, Tom L., 84

Blackstone, Sir William, 126, 128

Blustein, Jeffrey, 127, 129

Brecht, Bertolt, 45

Brock, Dan, 85-86

Brody, Elaine M., 122-23

Brody, Howard, 118, 205-9

Buchan, William, 6

Buchanan, Alan, 85-86

in, 205-9; preserving moral nature of, 210

Egg. *See* gamete
Elbaum: court case, 98-99
Emanuel, Ezekiel J., 90-92
Emanuel, Linda L., 88, 90-92
Embryo: creation of through IVF, 168; donation of, 166; frozen, 168-72; in *Davis* case, 169-77; "Is Mr. Davis Already a Father?" 169-70
Emerson, Ralph Waldo, 9
Ethics: at end of life, 149-54; impersonal, 55-56, of adoption, 159-61; of assisted suicide, 152-54; of care, 138; of caring for elderly, 125-33; of contract pregnancy, 163-67; of deception, 200, 204; of familial decisionmaking, 106-18; of familial resource allocation, 201-3; of families, 113; of favoritism, 186-99; of frozen embryos, 168-72; of genetic screening, 178-79; of intimacy, 63-82; of medicine, 56, 60-63, 113; of multiculturalism, 219-29; of respect for persons, 137-38, 145; of sperm vending, 161-63; patient-centered, 2-3, 26, 62-63, 117; reproductive, 155-80; theories of, 57-60; strategic, 226; universalizability of, 59-60

Family: abolition of, 33; and assisted suicide, 152-54; and justice, 181-93, 195-204, 209-18; and live donation of organs, 187-88, 213-14; and maintenance of self, 45-49; 148, 227; and reproduction, 155-80; and resource allocation, 201-3; and trust of professional caregivers, 217; archaic features of, 72; as conduit to patient's culture, 219-29; as caregivers for elderly, 121; as *Gesellschaft* or *Gemeinschaft*, 116-17; definition of, 31-35; demands on medicine of, 214-17; discussions in, 198; disownment in, 101, 164, 175; divorce in, 15, 22-23, 24-25, 192-93, 196; ethics of, 63-82; favoritism in, 64-67; functions of, 36-37, 86, 159-60; gender roles in, 9, 17, 21; history of, 8-9, 15-17, 21-25; "The Hospital Visitor's Policy," 52-53; liberalized, 197; neglected by bioethicists, 84-86; poverty in, 24; reform of, 186; romantic and cynical views of, 31-34, 139, 175; screening prospective members of, 178-79; sentimental model of, 8-9, 17, 22
Farquhar, George, 8
Father: abusive behavior of, 38; abandonment of children of, 162-63; and artificial insemination by vendor, 165; decision to be, 170; gay, 165-66; parental responsibility of, 183; relationship with child of, 108
Faulkner, William, 43
Feinberg, Joel, 127
Feminism: and abortion, 105-6; and burden of familial care, 113, 183, 184-85, 212; and conflict with multiculturalism, 228; and elder care, 122-23; and *Davis* case, 170-72; and families, 192-93; and lesbian separatist families, 165-66; and sexism in medicine, 194-95; and women in the workforce, 23; "Another Woman in the Middle," 183
Futility: "Helga Wanglie's Ventilator," 142-43; of sustaining patients in PVS, 4, 143-35, 216; medical, 216, 224

Gamete: retrieval of, 170-71; use of in IVF, 168; vending of egg, 166; vending of sperm, 161-63
Geach, Peter, 79
Genes: and genetic screening, 173-79; meaning of, 180; use of to determine parenthood, 167
Godwin, William, 66-67